KEY TOPICS IN
ONCOLOGY

The KEY TOPICS Series

Advisors:

T.M. Craft *Department of Anaesthesia and Intensive Care, Royal United Hospital, Bath, UK*
C.S. Garrard *Intensive Therapy Unit, John Radcliffe Hospital, Oxford, UK*
P.M. Upton *Department of Anaesthetics, Treliske Hospital, Truro, UK*

Anaesthesia, Second Edition

Obstetrics and Gynaecology

Accident and Emergency Medicine

Paediatrics

Orthopaedic Surgery

Otolaryngology and Head and Neck Surgery

Ophthalmology

Psychiatry

General Surgery

Renal Medicine

Chronic Pain

Trauma

Oral and Maxillofacial Surgery

Oncology

Forthcoming titles include:

Obstetrics and Gynaecology, Second Edition

Cardiovascular Medicine

Neonatology

Critical Care

Orthopaedic Trauma Surgery

Respiratory Medicine

Thoracic Surgery

KEY TOPICS IN
ONCOLOGY

G.D. HALL
MRCP(UK)

*ICRF Clinical Research Fellow and Honorary Registrar, ICRF Cancer
Medicine Research Unit, St James's University Hospital, Leeds, UK*

P.M. PATEL
PhD MRCP(UK)

*ICRF Clinical Scientist, Honorary Consultant in Medical Oncology,
ICRF Cancer Medicine Research Unit, St James's University Hospital,
Leeds, UK*

A.S. PROTHEROE
MRCP(UK)

*Lecturer in Medical Oncology, ICRF Cancer Medicine Research Unit,
St James's University Hospital, Leeds, UK*

Consultant Editor

P.J. SELBY
MA, MD, FRCP, FRCR

*Professor of Cancer Medicine, St. James's University Hospital,
Leeds, UK*

βIOS
SCIENTIFIC
PUBLISHERS

A CIP catalogue record for this book is available from the British Library.

ISBN 1 85996 105 3

BIOS Scientific Publishers Ltd
9 Newtec Place, Magdalen Road, Oxford OX4 1RE, UK
Tel. +44 (0)1865 726286. Fax. +44 (0)1865 246823
World Wide Web home page: http://www.Bookshop.co.uk/BIOS/

DISTRIBUTORS

Australia and New Zealand
    Blackwell Science Asia
    54 University Street
    Carlton, South Victoria 3053

India
    Viva Books Private Limited
    4325/3 Ansari Road, Daryaganj
    New Delhi 110002

Singapore and South East Asia
    Toppan Company (S) PTE Ltd
    38 Liu Fang Road, Jurong
    Singapore 2262

USA and Canada
    BIOS Scientific Publishers
    PO Box 605, Herndon
    VA 20172-0605

Important Note from the Publisher
The information contained within this book was obtained by BIOS Scientific Publishers Ltd from sources believed by us to be reliable. However, while every effort has been made to ensure its accuracy, no responsibility for loss or injury whatsoever occasioned to any person acting or refraining from action as a result of information contained herein can be accepted by the authors or publishers.

The reader should remember that medicine is a constantly evolving science and while the authors and publishers have ensured that all dosages, applications and practices are based on current indications, there may be specific practices which differ between communities. You should always follow the guidelines laid down by the manufacturers of specific products and the relevant authorities in the country in which you are practising.

Typeset by Chandos Electronic Publishing, Stanton Harcourt, UK.
Printed by Redwood Books, Trowbridge, UK.

CONTENTS

[a]Contributed by J. Chester, Specialist Registrar in Medical Oncology, St. James's University Hospital, Leeds, UK

[b]Contributed by D. Wyld, Medical Oncologist, Royal Brisbane Hospital, Brisbane, Australia

[c]Contributed by N. Spencer, Consultant Radiologist, Pindersfield's General Hospital, Wakefield, UK

[d]Contributed by J. Adams, Specialist Registrar in Medical Oncology, St. James's University Hospital, Leeds, UK

[e]Contributed by S. Cheeseman, Specialist Registrar in Medical Oncology, Christie Hospital, Manchester, UK

[f]Contributed by D. Jackson, Specialist Registar in Medical Oncology, St. James's University Hospital, Leeds, UK

[g]Contributed by D. Stark, Specialist Registrar in Medical Oncology, St. James's University Hospital, Leeds, UK

[h]Contributed by M. Stockton, Senior Registrar in Palliative Medicine, St. Gemma's Hospice, Leeds, UK

[i]Contributed by J. Ellis, Specialist Registrar in Paediatrics, St. James's University Hospital, Leeds, UK

[j]Contributed by M. Bennett, Consultant in Palliative Care, St. Gemma's Hospice, Leeds, UK

[k]Contributed by G. Velikova, Senior Registrar in Medical Oncology, St. James's University Hospital, Leeds, UK

[l]Contributed by J. Wylie, Specialist Registrar in Clinical Oncology, Christie Hospital, Manchester, UK

[m]Contributed by J. Howell, Royal Infirmary, Glasgow, UK

ABBREVIATIONS

βHCG	β human chorionic gonadotrophin
5-FU	5-fluorouracil
5-HT3	5-hydroxytryptamine
6-MP	6-mercaptopurine
ABVD	adriamycin/bleomycin/vinblastine/dacarbazine
AC	doxorubicin (adriamycin)/cyclophosphamide
ACTH	adrenocorticotrophic hormone
ADA	adenosine deaminase
ADCC	antibody-dependent cell mediated cytotoxicity
ADH	anti-diuretic hormone
AFP	α-fetoprotein
ALL	acute lymphoblastic leukaemia
AML	acute myeloblastic leukaemia
ATRA	all-*trans* retinoic acid
BCG	bacillus Calmette–Guérin
BCNU	carmustine
bd	twice daily
BEAM	carmustine/etoposide/cytarabine/melphalan
BMG	benign monoclonal gammopathy
BOLD	BCNU/vincristine/lomustine/DTIC
CAP	cisplatin/adriamycin/cyclophosphamide
CBV	cyclophosphamide/carmustine/etoposide
CCNU	Lomustine
Cdk	cyclin-dependent kinase
CEA	carcino-embryonic antigen
Ch1VPP	chlorambucil/vinblastine/procarbazine/prednisolone
CHOP	cyclophosphamide/doxorubicin/vincristine/prednisolone
CIN	cervical intraepithelial neoplasia
CKI	cyclin-dependent kinase inhibitor
CMF	cyclophosphamide/methotrexate/5-FU
CML	chronic myeloid leukaemia
CMV	cytomegalovirus
CNS	central nervous system
CSF	cerebral spinal fluid
CT	computed tomography
CTL	cytotoxic T lymphocyte
CTZ	chemoreceptor trigger zone
CVA	cerebrovascular accident
CVD	cisplatin/vinblastine/DTIC
CXR	chest X-ray

DIC	disseminated intravascular coagulation
DTIC	dacarbazine
DVT	deep venous thrombosis
EBV	Epstein–Barr virus
EBNA	Epstein–Barr nuclear antigens
ER	oestrogen receptor
ERCP	endoscopic retrograde cholangiopancreatography
FAB	French–American classification
FAC	5-FU/doxorubicin/cyclophosphamide
FBC	full blood count
FEC	5-FU/epirubicin/cyclophosphamide
FIGO	International Federation of Gynaecologists and Obstetricians
FNAC	fine-needle aspiration cytology
G-CSF	granulocyte-colony-stimulating factor
GI	gastrointestinal
GCP	good clinical practice
GM-CSF	granulocyte-macrophage-colony-stimulating growth factor
GVHD	graft-versus-host disease
HAMA	human-against-mouse antibodies
HCC	hepatocellular carcinoma
HIV	human immunodeficiency virus
HLA	human leukocyte antigen
HNPCC	hereditary non-polyposis colorectal carcinoma
HPOA	hypertrophic pulmonary osteoarthropathy
HPV	human papilloma virus
HSVTR	herpes simplex thymidine kinase
HTLV-1	human T-cell leukaemia type 1
Ig	immunoglobulin
IgH	immunoglobulin heavy chain
IFN-γ	interferon-γ
IFN-α	interferon-α
IL-2	interleukin-2
IM	intramuscular
IV	intravenous
LAK cell	lymphokine-activated killer cell
LD	lethal dose
LDH	lactate dehydrogenase
LEMS	Lambert–Eaton myasthenic syndrome
LHRH	lutenizing-hormone releasing hormone
MALT	mucosal-associated lymphoid tissue
M-VAC	methotrexate/vinblastine/adriamycin/cisplatin
M3G	morphine-3-glucuronide
M6G	morphine-6-glucuronide

MDR	multi-drug resistance
MEN	multiple endocrine neoplasia
MIBG	meta-iodobenzylguanidine
MMM	methotrexate/mitomycin C/mitozantrone
MRC	Medical Research Council
MRI	magnetic resonance imaging
MTD	maximum tolerated dose
NHL	non-Hodgkin's lymphoma
NK cell	natural killer cell
NSAIDs	non-steroidal anti-inflammatory drugs
NSCLC	non-small cell lung cancer
NSE	neuron-specific enolase
PBC	primary biliary cirrhosis
PCI	prophylactic cranial irradiation
PCP	pneumonocystis pneumonia
PCR	polymerase chain reaction
PCV	procarbazine/CCNU/vincristine
PET	positron emission tomography
Pgp	P-glycoprotein
PNET	primitive neuro-ectodermal tumour
pRb	retinoblastoma protein
PSA	prostate-specific antigen
Rb	retinoblastoma
RCC	renal cell carcinoma
REAL	revised European–American lymphoma
S/C	subcutaneously
SCLC	small-cell lung cancer
SVCO	superior vena cava obstruction
QL	quality of life
QUASAR	quick and simple and reliable
TNF	tumour necrosis factor
TNM	primary tumour, associated nodal disease and distant metastases
TS	thymidylate synthetase
TSA	tumour-specific antigen
TSH	thyroid-stimulating hormone
VMA	vanillylmandelic acid
WHO	World Health Organization

PREFACE

One in three people will develop cancer during their lifetime. Cancer medicine is therefore relevant to all disciplines of medicine from general practise to hospital specialities. This book covers a range of topics central to cancer practise including basic science, surgery, radiotherapy, chemotherapy and palliative care. This reflects an attempt to emphasize the integrated approach essential for the optimal management of patients with cancer.

This book will be of value to all medical professionals including registrars in oncology and other specialities, general practitioners, nursing staff and undergraduates. It should be particularly useful for candidates studying for postgraduate exams such as the MRCP.

We would like to thank BIOS for their help and patience in preparing this book.

G.D. Hall
P.M. Patel
A.S. Protheroe

AETIOLOGICAL AGENTS

For most cancers the cause of the initial malignant changes remain unclear. Aetiological agents have been identified for some cancers, for example cigarette smoking and lung cancer, Epstein–Barr virus (EBV) and Burkitt's lymphoma, and radiation and the leukaemias. These causative agents have been linked predominantly by epidemiological studies. The mechanisms by which these agents exert their effect are being increasingly unravelled. For many cancers a combination of several agents may be necessary, allowing an accumulation of genetic aberrations that leads to a malignant phenotype.

Many classes of aetiological agent are recognized. These include:

Familial
Inherited conditions, characterized by specific genetic defects, are associated with an increased risk of one or more cancers. A germline deletion of one allele of a gene and subsequent mutation of the remaining allele leads to carcinogenesis. Examples include neurofibromatosis, adenomatous polyposis coli, familial breast cancer and von-Hippel Lindau syndrome. The identification of the specific genetic defect in familial cancer frequently leads to the identification of genes important in the pathogenesis of related acquired tumours.

Chemicals
Many chemicals act as carcinogens by damaging cellular DNA and inducing mutations in oncogenes and tumour suppressor genes. Carcinogenic chemicals include:

- Cigarette smoke – carcinogens present in cigarette smoke causes specific mutations in the *p53* tumour-suppressor gene.
- Aromatic amines – associated with bladder cancer.
- Benzene – leukaemia.
- Wood dust – nasal adenocarcinoma.
- Vinyl chloride – angiosarcomas.

Physical
Radiation. This increases the risk of cancer by increasing DNA damage leading to the accumulation of mutations in tumour-suppressor genes and oncogenes. The risk of tumour development is associated with:

- Radiation source – high-energy radiation (α-particles) is more carcinogenic than lower energy

X-rays or γ-rays from a cobalt source. Damage to DNA by UV light is pathogenic in skin cancers, including malignant melanoma.

- Level of exposure – the dose received is critical to the incidence of tumour development. Accumulation of the radioactive isotope in a particular tissue may lead to tumour formation, for example thyroid cancer and radioactive iodine.

Infective

Infective agents which are associated with cancer include:

1. Human papilloma virus (HPV). The E6 protein produced by HPV16 binds to and inactivates the p53 protein. This leads to dysregulation of the cell cycle and apoptotic pathways and subsequent malignant transformation of epithelial cells infected. Cervical and anal cancer are associated with sexual transmission of HPV.

2. Epstein–Barr virus. Infection is associated with non-Hodgkin's lymphoma (NHL) and other lymphomas. The most common genetic abnormality, a 14:8 translocation in which the proto-oncogene c-myc on chromosome 8 becomes transcriptionally controlled by the control elements of immunoglobulin genes on chromosome 14, is thought to be caused by Epstein–Barr nuclear antigens (EBNA).

3. Hepatitis B virus. Infection is associated with hepatocellular cancer and leads to a greater than 100-fold increased risk.

4. Retrovirus. By integration into the cellular genome retroviruses can cause abnormal overexpression of oncogenes. Retroviral infection has been implicated in numerous animal tumours. In humans, HTLV1 infection is associated with T-cell lymphomas.

5. Helicobacter pylori. This has recently been identified as a causative factor in malignancy, particularly in mucosal associated lymphoid tissue (MALT) tumours. Eradication of the *H. pylori* may lead to a regression of the tumour.

Diet Many differing food substances have been implicated as causative agents through demographic studies, for example the association of colorectal carcinomas with low-fibre diets (as in the Western world) and gastric carcinomas with smoked food (as in Japan). Many of the carcinogens are breakdown products of food, for example nitrosamines. Low-fibre diets lead to a decrease of transit time through the bowel, thereby increasing exposure to carcinogenic substances.

Immune deficiencies There is increasing evidence that the immune system is involved in tumour surveillance. Drugs causing immunodeficiency are associated with a higher risk of malignancy, as are infections that damage the immune system, for example HIV. Congenital abnormalities of the immune system, particularly T-cell deficiencies, are also associated with an increased risk of tumours.

Drugs Cytotoxic drugs induce DNA damage and are associated with an increased risk of malignancy. The effect is dose dependent and therefore of considerable importance in high-dose regimes. Characteristic translocations may be induced by the topoisomerase inhibitors and lead to an acute leukaemia.

Further reading

Peckham M, Priedo H, Veroneri U. *Oxford Textbook of Oncology,* Oxford University Press, 1995.

Related topics of interest

Familial cancer syndromes (p. 92)
Smoking (p. 241)

APOPTOSIS

Cell death occurs by either necrosis or apoptosis. Necrosis follows physical damage to a cell that leads to disruption of the cell membrane and hence loss of cell viability. By contrast, apoptosis is an active cellular process that leads to degradation of the cellular DNA and subsequent cell death. This process is under tight cellular control in response to specific stimuli. Apoptosis is often referred to as programmed cell death.

Apoptosis is a normal process essential to embryonic development and the maintenance of normal cell numbers in adult tissues. Different tissues undergo apoptosis at different rates. More than 95% of lymphocytes and 75% of spermatocytes produced are believed to undergo apoptosis. Apoptosis is also induced in cells that are abnormal.

Apoptotic cell death

Appearance

Cells dying by apoptosis have a characteristic appearance. They initially lose contact with neighbouring cells and shrink. The formation of cytoplasmic blebs (apoptotic bodies), the condensation of chromatin and the fragmentation of nuclear DNA into 200 base pair fragments is followed by cell disruption. Phagocytosis of the cell debris by surrounding cells occurs rapidly, preventing an inflammatory response and subsequent damage to surrounding cells. The absence of an inflammatory response is a key difference between apoptosis and necrosis.

Apoptotic pathway

A basic biochemical pathway has been identified which appears to result in apoptotic cell death from a wide variety of signals. The common effector pathway is driven by the activity of caspases, a family of enzymes (cysyteine proteases), of which interleukin 1β converting enzyme was the first identified. Caspase activation leads to activation of numerous enzymatic pathways, leading to the morphological characteristics described.

Apoptotic control

The apoptosis pathway is under strict cellular regulation to ensure that activation occurs only under appropriate conditions. A family of proteins has been identified which is involved in regulating the process. The first discovered bcl-2, was originally isolated in B-cell lymphoma where overexpression of the protein results from the 14:18 translocation, following which the *bcl-2* gene (chromosome 18) is placed under the control of the immunoglobulin heavy-chain promoter on chromosome 14. bcl-2 overexpression in B cells prolongs their survival and subsequently leads to tumourigenesis.

A number of bcl-2 family members have been identified (bax, bak, bcl-X and Bad) which form dimers with other family members (heterodimers) or themselves (homodimers). Bax induces apoptosis whereas bcl-2 protects cells. It is currently proposed that bcl-2 and other family members compete for the binding of Bax in order to inactivate it and prevent apoptosis.

Apoptotic signals

A variety of signals lead to apoptosis. These may be extracellular or intracellular in origin.

1. Extracellular signals. Activation of a receptor molecule Fas by its associated ligand leads to apoptosis through the TNF signalling pathway. This mechanism of activation is the key signal in the apoptosis of activated lymphocytes. Loss of cell–cell contact or loss of growth signals may also activate apoptosis.

2. Intracellular signals. The detection of DNA damage, such as double-strand breaks, activates apoptosis in most cells. p53 increases transcription of *bax* and represses transcription of bcl-2, thereby altering the balance of these regulators in favour of apoptosis. p53-independant responses to DNA damage have also been identified.

Apoptosis and disease

Abnormalities in the regulation of apoptosis contribute to the pathogenesis of a wide range of diseases.

Decreased apoptosis

An inhibition of apoptosis with inappropriate cell proliferation is believed to be central to the pathogenesis of:

- Cancer.
- Autoimmune disease.
- Viral infection.

Increased apoptosis Increased apoptosis with inadequate cell proliferation is associated with:

- AIDS, leading to depletion of CD4$^+$ lymphocytes.
- Neurodegenerative disorders, e.g. Parkinson's disease.
- Myelodysplastic syndromes.

Apoptosis and cancer

Apoptotic failure DNA damage, with loss of tumour-supressor-gene expression and overexpression of oncogenes, is central to neoplastic transformation and the development of cancer. In normal cells such DNA damage is a powerful stimulus to apoptosis. Knowledge of how cancer cells evade apoptotic death is therefore central to understanding tumour development.

The failure of the pathogenic DNA damage to initiate apoptosis also brings into question the wisdom of treating cancer with agents designed to induce DNA damage.

Apoptosis therapeutics Reactivation of the apoptotic response to DNA damage is an attractive mechanism for treating cancer and the focus of much molecular research.

Further reading

Thompson CB. Apoptosis in the pathogenesis and treatment of disease. *Science*, 1995; **267:** 1456–62.
Nagata S. Apoptosis by death factor. *Cell*, 1997; **88:** 355–65.

Related topics of interest

Cell cycle (p. 40)
Molecular biology of cancer (p. 151)

BIOLOGICAL THERAPY

The broadest definition of biological therapies includes the use of agents that are normally found in the body and exert a biological effect. This includes hormones, cytokines, growth factors and antibodies. Some definitions include immunotherapies such as vaccines.

Cytokines

Cytokines are protein molecules secreted by cells that regulate the immune and inflammatory responses. Nomenclature does not necessarily pertain to biological function. Cytokines used in clinical practice include the interferons, the interleukins and several other growth factors. Most exert differing effects on different cell types. The most commonly used cytokines are:

Interferons

Two classes exist: α and β interferons (class I) and γ interferon (class II). Both play a role in the immune response to viruses but also have anti-tumour effects. The anti-tumour effects are either direct by exerting an anti-proliferative response or indirect by enhancing host immune response.

α and β interferons can be secreted by most cell types in response to viral infection. The presence of double-stranded viral RNA induces their secretion. These cytokines exert a direct anti-proliferative effect on several cell types including cancer cell lines. In addition, they induce the expression of major histocompatability complex (MHC) molecules which increase antigen presentation.

Interferons can be administered IV, IM or S/C. Systemic interferon has anti-tumour effect in hairy cell leukaemia, CML and multiple myeloma. In these situations interferon can significantly increase the length of remissions induced by other agents. Interferon alone has a 15% response rate in renal cancer and its role in combination with other biological agents is being investigated. The role of adjuvant interferon is being investigated in high-risk melanoma but early trials have shown a beneficial effect.

The main side effects of interferon are flu-like symptoms of fever and rigors and lethargy. The former improve with repeated injection and the latter accumulates. At higher doses hepatotoxicity and myelosuppression can occur.

Interleukins

Interleukins have a predominantly immunological role. IL-2 is the most studied interleukin in the clinical context. Newer cytokines are being investigated and include IL-12, which has a role in enhancing cell-mediated cytotoxicity. Other interleukins may also potentially be of use in cancer treatments (IL-15, IL-18, IL-20).

The use of combination biological and chemotherapy is being investigated. In renal cancer and melanoma phase II studies show increased response rates and some studies suggest that biological agents may increase the number and length of remissions in selected patients.

Haematopoetic growth factors

Granulocyte-colony-stimulating growth factors (G-CSF) and Granulocyte-macrophage-colony-stimulating growth factors (GM-CSF) are cytokines that promote proliferation and differentiation of haematopoetic progenitor cells.

When administered systemically (by S/C injection daily) these growth factors increase recovery of neutrophil counts following chemotherapy. They are therefore useful in the treatment of prolonged neutropenias, or in allowing more dose-intensive myelosuppressive chemotherapy. In addition, G-CSF and GM-CSF promote the release of haematopoetic stem cells into the circulation and therefore are used for stem cell mobilization enabling peripheral blood stem cell harvesting prior to high-dose chemotherapy.

Hormones

Several tumours are known to be influenced by hormones, including breast cancer, uterine cancer and prostate cancer.

Breast cancer

A large proportion of breast cancer cells have oestrogen receptors and blocking the oestrogen effect can significantly reduce tumour activity. This is possible either by reducing endogenous oestrogen (by drug or oophrectomy) or by blocking the receptor. The following anti-oestrogens are used:

1. Tamoxifen. This binds the oestrogen receptor. Tamoxifen reduces the relapse rate after breast surgery in post-menopausal women and can have a significant antitumour effect in advanced disease.

2. Aromatase inhibitors. These inhibit the production of oestrodiol from its precursors estriol and eastrone. Agents in this class include aminoglutethamide, formestane and anastrazole.

3. Progestogens. These include medroxyprogesterone and megesterol.

Prostate cancer

Similarly, around 80% of prostate cancers are androgen-dependent so orchidectomy or anti-androgenic agents can be used as treatment.

Anti-androgen therapy is used in prostate cancer. Agents can act at several points in the pituitary, adrenal, testicular axis.

1. Cytopoterone acetate. This blocks activity at the target tissues and also has a pituitary affect. It is often used first line in advanced prostate cancer.

2. Flutamide. This also blocks androgen activity at the target tissues and can be used instead of cypoterone acetate.

3. GnRH analogues. These include goserelin, which results in reduced androgen production. It is given monthly depot injections.

To achieve complete androgen blockade two agents may be combined.

Antibodies

Infusion of antibodies directed against tumours has been tried for several cancers including breast cancer, lymphomas and colorectal cancer. Antibodies can be given either alone, the aim here being to mobilize host antibody dependent cellular cytotoxicty (ADCC) mechanisms, or conjugated to toxins such as ricin or radioactive moieties. Earlier studies used mouse monoclonal antibodies. These, however, induced human-against-mouse antibodies (HAMA), hence reducing efficacy and preventing repeated injections. Recombinant technology has allowed the production of humanized antibodies which reduce this effect.

To date, the use of antibody-mediated therapy is experimental, but has shown promise in some areas, for example the Panorex antibody against colorectal cancer may reduce relapse in Dukes'-C colorectal cancer and anti-B-cell antibodies in non-Hodgkin's lymphoma.

Miscellaneous

Other therapies which can be considered under biological treatments and which are for the most part still experimental include the following.

Donor leukocyte infusions	This method can be used to treat relapses following allogeneic transplantation in CML. Leukocytes have also been used that are specific for viral infections (CMV/EBV) post-transplantation.
Peptides	Clinical trials are studying the effect of vaccinating patients with peptides specific for tumour antigens, in the hope of inducing a host response to the malignancy.
Dendritic cells	Patients are being vaccinated with dendritic cells (professional antigen presenting cells) loaded with tumour antigens, in the hope of better presentation of tumour peptides.

Further reading

DeVita VT, Hellman S, Rosenberg SA. *Biological Theory of Cancer,* 2nd edn. Philadelphia: JB Lippincott.

Related topics of interest

BLADDER CANCER

Background

Incidence

Bladder cancer has an incidence of approximately 13 000 in the UK. It is more common in males than females with a male to female ratio of approximately 2.5:1. It is the fourth most common malignancy in males and the tenth most common malignancy in females.

Risk factors

1. Smoking. The risk of bladder cancer correlates with both the duration of smoking and the number of cigarettes smoked. It accounts for half of the cases among men and about one third among women.

2. Industrial carcinogens. Exposure to aromatic amines, particularly 2-napthylamine and benzidine and their analogues is associated with an increased risk. Exposure to these chemicals is common in the dye, chemical, rubber, leather, paint and aluminium industries.

3. Drugs. Phenacetin, an analgesic in general use 20 years ago, is associated with tumours of the renal tract. Cytotoxic drugs, especially cyclophosphamide, have been linked to an increased risk of bladder cancer.

4. Schistosomiasis. Infestation with *Schistosoma haematobium* is associated with a higher incidence of squamous cell carcinoma of the bladder.

Aetiology

Specific chromosomal abnormalities have been identified in bladder cancer with non-random changes of chromosomes 1, 5, 7, 9, 11 and 17 recognized. Oncogenes such as *ras* and *c-erb-B2* are activated; tumour-suppressor genes *p53* and *Rb-1* are inactivated. *p53* inactivation has been linked to the ability of a bladder cancer to become invasive.

Histology

Bladder cancer arises from the urothelium which lines the renal tract from the renal pelvis to the urethra.

Transitional cell carcinoma. These constitute more than 90% of all tumours. Tumours are described morphologically (papillary and non-papillary), by level of invasion and by histological grade.

More than two thirds present as non-invasive papillary tumours. The majority of these are well differentiated (grade 1) which rarely become invasive (10% in a 10 year follow-up). Multiple lesions occur in approximately 50% of patients.

Carcinoma *in situ* has traditionally been considered with other superficial non-invasive lesions. However, its behaviour is highly aggressive, with approximately 50% progressing to muscle invasion, and it must be considered a high-risk lesion.

Non-papillary transitional cell carcinomas are less common and usually of at least grade 3 histology. They are associated with frequent progression to muscle invasion.

Others. Squamous carcinoma, adenocarcinoma and neuroendocrine tumours are recognized but infrequent.

Clinical features

Presentation

Urinary symptoms such as haematuria, frequency, urgency and dysuria are the most common symptoms of early bladder cancer. Other symptoms (e.g. pelvic pain, bone pain, urinary obstruction,) usually occur late as the result of invasive or metastatic disease.

Investigations

Urinalysis. Cytological analysis should be performed on a fresh urine specimen. Positive cytology is found in 90% of poorly differentiated tumours; less than 50% of well differentiated lesions are positive. Carcinoma *in situ* gives positive cytology in almost 100% of cases.

Cystoscopy. This enables detailed visual inspection of all areas of the bladder. Biopsies of all abnormal areas should be taken and should include the base of the tumour to allow assessment of muscle invasion. Adjacent and distant mucosa should also be biopsied.

Intravenous urography. An excretory urogram will demonstrate the presence of lesions within the renal pelvis and ureters. Ureteric obstruction usually implying invasive disease can also be visualized.

Ultrasound. In combination with urine cytology, ultrasound may effectively diagnose superficial bladder tumours. Its sensitivity for tumours in the upper renal tract is poor.

CT scanning. Muscle invasive tumours should be fully assessed for evidence of metastatic disease. The use of CT in addition to transurethral biopsy and bimanual examination improves the accuracy of staging.

Staging

Bladder cancer is most commonly staged using the TNM classification.

Tx	Primary tumour cannot be assessed.
T0	No evidence of primary tumour.
Tis	Carcinoma *in situ*.
Ta	Non-invasive papillary tumour.
T1	Tumour invades subepithelial connective tissue.
T2	Tumour invades superficial muscle.
T3	Tumour invades deep muscle or perivesical fat.
T4	Tumour invades adjacent organs.
N0	No evidence of regional lymph nodes.
N1	Single lymph node less than 2 cm.
N2	Single lymph node 2–5 cm in diameter or multiple lymph nodes less than 5 cm.
N3	Lymph node(s) greater than 5 cm.
M0	No distant metastases.
M1	Distant metastases present.

Management of superficial carcinoma (Ta, T1 and Tis)

Surgery

Trans-urethral resection of all lesions by rigid cystoscopy is required. Diathermy of lesions is not recommended as histological assessment of all lesions should ideally be performed. The risk of tumour recurrence is up to 80% and therefore regular cystoscopy may be needed.

Disease at high risk of progression (extensive carcinoma *in situ*, multiple high grade lesions) may be managed with bladder resection.

Intravesical therapy

Single, low grade, Ta tumours seldom recur following destruction and therefore no further treatment is required. However, patients with multiple, recurrent or high-risk lesions (invasive (T1) lesions or carcinoma *in situ*) should receive additional intravesical therapy.

Chemotherapy. Mitomycin C, thiotepa or epirubicin administered at cystoscopy reduce tumour recurrence.

The ability of intravesical chemotherapy to reduce progression to muscle invasion is less well defined. Mitomycin C is not absorbed by the bladder and therefore systemic toxicity is minimal.

Immunotherapy. The administration of intravesical BCG (bacillus Calmette-Guérin) stimulates a local immune response which reduces both the rate of local recurrence and progression. Intravesical BCG induces local toxicity such as cystitis (90%) in addition fever, malaise and nausea. Intravesical BCG is the most effective topical therapy for carcinoma *in situ*.

Management of invasive disease

Surgery

In a small proportion of patients, trans-urethral resection of superficial invasive disease may be appropriate. Partial or total cystectomy is required for more advanced disease. Urinary diversion, most frequently with an ileal conduit, is also required.

Cystectomy alone may be curative for disease confined to the bladder. However, additional treatment with chemotherapy or radiotherapy is frequently employed.

Urinary diversion may also be employed in the palliative setting.

Radiotherapy

Radical radiotherapy may be as effective as cystectomy. This enables the morbidity of a cystectomy to be avoided. Neoadjuvant radiotherapy may downstage a tumour, making it operable. Radiotherapy may be given as external beam therapy and/or brachytherapy. Radiotherapy may induce haematuria and eventually lead to a fibrosed shrunken bladder. However, the rate of impotence is significantly lower than that following radical cystectomy.

Radiotherapy to palliate locally advanced, inoperable disease may also be used to control symptoms.

Chemotherapy

Cisplatin, methotrexate, vinblastine and adriamycin are the most active and therefore most frequently employed chemotherapy agents. As single agents, response rates from 15–40% are achieved. Combination chemotherapy with cisplatin, methotrexate and vinblastine with or without doxorubicin (adriamycin) [cisplatin/ methotrexate/vinblastine or methotrexate/vinblastine/ adriamycin/cisplatin (M-VAC)] increase both the overall and complete response rates (40–70% and 15–35% respectively).

Squamous and adenocarcinoma are generally unresponsive to chemotherapy.

Combination therapy

Despite apparent curative surgery or radical radiotherapy many patients die from distant metastases. This has led to the combination of modalities to provide optimal local control with surgery or radiotherapy and adjuvant chemotherapy to prevent distant relapse.

Prognostic factors

Stage of tumour

The depth of muscle invasion and the degree of differentiation are the most important prognostic factors. Following radical cystectomy, tumours with invasion confined to superficial muscle (T1 or T2) are associated with 5 year progression-free survival of between 50 and 70%. Those with deeper invasion (T3) have a 20–40% 5 year progression-free survival. Five year survival in patients with more advanced disease is uncommon.

Age

Prognosis deteriorates with increasing age.

| **p53** | Although not routinely assessed, superficial tumours with *p53* abnormalities are associated with a worse prognosis. |

Current issues

Molecular prognostics	Genetic factors which predict for the progression of superficial tumours to muscle invasion, may identify patients who need more aggressive therapy for superficial disease.
Combination therapy	The optimal combination of surgery, radiotherapy and chemotherapy is not clear. Recent studies of neoadjuvant chemotherapy prior to surgery or radiotherapy have been inconclusive. Further randomized studies are required.
New drugs	Taxanes have been demonstrated to have high activity against bladder tumours. Their incorporation into standard regimes is being investigated.

Further reading

Ozen, H. Bladder cancer. *Current Opinion in Oncology,* 1997; **9:** 295–300.

BONE CANCER

Background

Incidence

Primary bone tumours are rare with approximately 500 new cases occurring in the UK each year. Overall, there is a slightly higher incidence in males than in females. The different types of bone primaries vary in age distribution. The common types occur most frequently in adolescents, probably reflecting the rapid rate of growth of bones at this stage.

Risk factors

No common aetiological agent has been identified. Osteosarcomas are associated with ionizing radiation. Certain pre-existing bone diseases predispose to the development of osteosarcoma and less commonly chondrosarcoma (e.g. Paget's disease).

Specific genetic defects have been linked to the pathogenesis of primary bone tumours. Genetic syndromes associated with loss of *p53* (Li–Fraumeni) or *Rb* (familial retinoblastoma) function are both associated with an increased incidence. Ewing's sarcoma is associated with a characteristic chromosomal translocation t(11:22).

Histology

Primary bone tumours may arise from any of the tissues which form bone.

- Osteogenic   Approx. 20%, e.g. osteosarcoma.
- Chondrogenic   Approx. 20 %, e.g. chondro-sarcoma.
- Fibrogenic   Approx. 4 %, e.g. fibrosarcoma.
- Unknown origin   Approx. 10%, e.g. Ewing's sarcoma.
- Haematopoietic   Approx. 40%, e.g. myeloma.

Osteosarcoma, Ewing's sarcoma and chondrosarcoma account for approximately 30% of all bone tumours (excluding haematopoietic).

The majority of malignant bone tumours are, however, secondaries from other primary tumours (especially from breast, bronchus, kidney, prostate and thyroid primaries).

Clinical features

Presentation

Osteosarcoma usually presents in adolescents and young adults. 45–60% arise in bones on either side of the knee joint, usually with painful swelling during a growth spurt. Others present following pathological fracture. Systemic features such as fever, anorexia or weight loss are rare. Metastases to other bones and to lungs are quite common, and may be manifest at presentation. Lymph node metastases are rare.

Ewing's sarcoma has a peak incidence between 10 and 20 years old, and occurs predominantly in the pelvis, femur and tibia. Painful swelling and tenderness are the most common features. Metastases to other bones and to lungs occur frequently.

Chondrosarcoma presents most frequently in middle age. The tumour is slow growing. It also presents with painful swelling in the pelvis, ribs and pectoral girdle. Metastases are infrequent and occur only with high-grade tumours.

Investigations

On plain films, all three common bone malignancies show destruction or erosion. In the case of osteosarcoma, new bone formation (giving 'sunray spicules') and periosteal elevation produce the appearance of Codman's triangle. Chondrosarcoma shows calcification of new bone as flecks rather than spicules, while periosteal reaction in Ewing's sarcoma results in an 'onion-skin' radiological appearance. In addition to plain-film radiographs of the affected region, CT or MRI can be helpful in assessing the extent of local spread.

Metastases to other bones and lungs from osteosarcoma and Ewing's sarcoma are frequent. Chest X-ray, CT and bone scans are required for complete staging.

Raised serum alkaline phosphatase can be a useful marker for osteosarcoma.

Patients with suspected tumours should be evaluated early by a specialist, as inappropriately performed biopsies might preclude subsequent limb sparing procedures.

Staging

Staging is defined on the degree of local spread. Histological grade is also an important prognostic indicator and thus also partly defines stage.

Stage I: low-grade A intra-compartmental spread only

                                 B extra-compartmental

Stage II: high-grade A intra-compartmental spread only

                                 B extra-compartmental

Stage III: regional or distant metastases (independent of grade local extent)

Management

Bone tumours require a multi-disciplinary approach in specialist centres. Improved surgical techniques have enabled more conservative surgery. Optimal treatment is different for the three main histological sub-types.

Osteosarcoma

Complete resection of the primary disease is required for curative management. The use of reconstructive surgery and prosthetic insertions has reduced the frequency of amputation. Adjuvant chemotherapy is an important component of treatment as pulmonary and bone metastases occur in most patients; its use dramatically improves long-term survival. Chemotherapy and surgery are often intercalated with combination chemotherapy (doxorubicin, ifosfamide or methotrexate-based) divided into 6–8 weeks prior to surgery and 10–20 weeks after. Pulmonary metastatic disease can also be treated by surgical removal prior to combination chemotherapy. Patients with bony metastases have a poor prognosis. Radiotherapy is used for local control where total surgical excision is not feasible, as in the pelvis, but response is often short term.

Ewing's sarcoma

Management principles are similar as for osteosarcoma with local control achieved with surgery or radiotherapy. Additional adjuvant chemotherapy improves the 5 year survival from 10–20% to 50–60%. Patients with metastatic disease are treated with local radiotherapy and combination chemotherapy.

| **Chondrosarcoma** | Surgical resection with control of local disease is the treatment of choice for chondrosarcoma, where early metastasis is rarer. Radiotherapy is used for inoperable tumours. Chrondosarcoma is less sensitive to chemotherapy and radiotherapy. |

Prognostic factors

| **Histology** | Overall 5 year survival figures are: |

- Osteosarcoma   60%.
- Ewing's sarcoma 50–60%.
- Chondrosarcoma 35%.

| **Stage** | Higher stages are associated with poorer survival. For Ewing's sarcoma, 5 year survival rates are 70% for tumour volume less than or equal to 500 ml and 75% for volume greater than 500 ml. |

Further reading

Jurgens H, Sauer R, Winkleman W, Goßel U. In: Peckham M, Priedo H, Veroneri U, eds. *Oxford Textbook of Oncology,* 2nd edn. Oxford University Press, 1995; 1953–60.

Souhami R, Cannon S. In: Peckham M, Priedo H, Veroneri U, eds. *Oxford Textbook of Oncology,* 2nd edn. Oxford University Press, 1995; 1960–76.

BRAIN TUMOURS

Background

Incidence

In the UK there are approximately 3000 new cases, and a similar number of deaths, each year. In most tumour types there is a slight male predominance. There is a bi-modal distribution, with peaks in the first decade of life [medulloblastomas and primitive neuro-ectodermal tumours (PNETs)], and at 40–60 years (glial cell tumours predominating).

Risk factors

Primary brain tumours show some marked associations:

- Neurofibrosarcoma – von Recklinghausen's disease.
- Gliomata – tuberose sclerosis.
- Cerebellar haemangioblastomata – von Hippel-Lindau syndrome.
- Embryonal cell tumour medulloblastoma – Gorlin's syndrome.

Aetiology

No clear aetiological agent has been identified for most primary tumours. Increasingly, a genetic pathogenesis has been identified: amplification of the proto-oncogenes *myc* and *ras* is seen in approximately 50% of glioblastoma multiforme cases. PNET may involve deletions in chromosome 17q; monosomy 22 is seen in up to 70% of meningiomata.

Histology

Primary tumours of the brain are subdivided according to the tissue of origin.

Glial cell tumours (gliomata). These account for just over half of all brain primaries, and over 90% of CNS primaries overall. There are four main categories of glioma:

- Astrocytomata – from the astrocyte population of supporting cells, these are the most common glial cell tumours.
- Oligodendroglioma – from the nutritive cells.
- Ependymoma – from the CSF-producing cells.
- PNETs – embryonal tumours.

Non-glial tumours. These include the following:

- Fibrous-tissue-derived (from the meninges), e.g. meningioma and meningiosarcoma, accounting for around 20% of brain tumours.
- Neuro-endocrine-derived tumours of the pituitary gland account for around 15%. Adenomatous tumours of the pituitary gland can be divided into tumours derived from the following.
  (a) Large chromophobe cells (50%).
  (b) Smaller chromophil cells – acidophils/ eosinophils (40%) and basophils (10%).
- Neurally-derived tumours (rare), e.g. acoustic neuromata.
- Suprasellar tumours, e.g. craniopharyngioma.
- Other rare brain primaries include those derived from the pineal, brain germ cell tumours, primary cerebral lymphoma, chordoma and vascular tumours.

Secondary tumours account for around one third of all brain tumours: the most common primaries are lung, breast and melanoma. Approximately 80% are intra-cranial tumours, and the rest extra-cranial (i.e. spinal cord), where they may be extra-dural or intra-dural.

Macroscopically, brain tumours rarely spread beyond the CNS, except for medulloblastoma which can metastasize to bone, and, less often, to lung and lymph nodes. Some cerebral tumours growing close to the mid-line can also spread across to the contralateral hemisphere via the corpus callosum.

Clinical features

Presentation

The clinical features of brain tumours can be subdivided:

Focal. Focal neurology can result, depending on the site of the tumour.

Generalized. This category includes the effects of raised intra-cranial pressure, caused either by local peri-tumour oedema or hydrocephalus secondary to tumour compression of the ventricular system. Symptoms include headaches, seizures and personality changes. Pituitary tumours may present as a result of a hormone secreted, for example galactorrhoea or amenorrhoea resulting from a prolactinoma.

Investigations

CT and MRI. These are the investigations of choice with the latter being particularly useful for posterior fossa and brain stem tumours. MRI is also useful for the diagnosis of spinal cord tumours.

Plain-film skull radiographs. These can identify tumours that calcify, for example craniopharyngioma, oligodendroglioma and some meningiomata.

Lumbar puncture. Cytological examination of CSF may show malignant tumour cells.

Visual field perimetry. This may confirm visual field defects associated with pituitary tumours.

Biochemical investigations. These may confirm the diagnosis of a 'functional' hormone-secreting pituitary tumour, with abnormally high levels of a particular hormone, such as prolactin, being present in the serum, or, less commonly assayed, the CSF.

Histological diagnosis. This is mandatory, for prognostic and therapeutic implications via radiologically-guided, or stereotactic biopsy. Open biopsy is rarely performed now.

Staging

There is no staging system in use.

Management

Supportive

In primaries with a particuarly bad prognosis, aggressive or invasive therapies such as surgery or combination chemotherapy may not be appropriate, and the main treatment options will be symptomatic, including:

1. Steroids (ususally dexamethasone). These are given as a treatment for peri-tumour oedema and raised intracranial pressure. A good response to steroids, which is usually rapid, often indicates a good response to subsequent radiotherapy.

2. Anti-convulsants. These may also provide important symptomatic relief.

3. Medical therapies. These can avoid the need for more aggressive treatment. For example the hormone antagonist bromocriptine is often a sufficient treatment for prolactinoma of the pituitary.

Surgery

Where aggressive therapy is appropriate, however, neurosurgery is the mainstay of treatment, not least because of the limited usefulness of radiotherapy and chemotherapy. Surgical removal should be as complete as possible while preserving neurological function.

Radiotherapy

Most neurological tumours (medulloblastoma being a notable exception) are radio-resistant. The main role for radiotherapy in primary brain tumours is as adjuvant post-operative therapy, to reduce the risk of local recurrence of higher grade tumours, or in lower grade tumours where incomplete surgical resection is suspected. Radiotherapy is more useful in the treatment of metastatic tumours where the primary is reasonably radiosensitive, such as small-cell carcinoma of the lung, or breast cancer.

Chemotherapy

Neither intravenous nor intrathecal chemotherapy are of widespread use in brain tumours. The only anti-tumour drugs with significant response rates are lipid-soluble drugs such as the nitrosureas (e.g. BCNU and CCNU) or very-high-dose methotrexate. Response rates of up to 40% for single agents can be obtained, with even higher rates for combination chemotherapy regimens such as PCV (procarbazine/CCNU/vincristine). Chemotherapy has a role in the treatment of germ cell tumours of the brain, or metastases from extra-CNS tumours such as small-cell lung cancer or testicular teratoma.

Prognostic factors

The prognosis for the CNS tumours is very variable.

Site

Generally the prognosis for intracranial tumours is worse than for spinal cord tumours, which tend to be of lower grade.

Histology

Slow-growing meningioma and cranio-pharyngioma have a 5 year overall survival of around 80%.

Grade

- Grade 1 astrocytoma approx. 60% 5 year survival.
- Grade 4 (glioblastoma multiforme) <10% 5 year survival.

One year survival is only approximately 30% and median survival only 3 months untreated or 8 months with radiotherapy for glioblastoma multiforme.

Other

Other poor prognostic indicators include increasing age, poor neurological performance status, incomplete surgical excision and the absence of epileptiform symptoms.

Further reading

Brada M, Thomas DGT. In: Peckham M, Priedo HM, Veroneri U, eds. *Oxford Textbook of Oncology,* 2nd edn. Oxford University Press, 1995; 2063–94.

Related topic of interest

Endocrine tumours (p. 84)

BREAKING BAD NEWS

Communication skills are not innate abilities that cannot be altered. There is now much research to show that effective communication skills consist of structures and concepts that can be learnt and improved. Effective skills enable better psychological adjustment by the patient, reduce stress in doctors and facilitate open, informed discussion between patients, their relatives and their doctors.

Bad news is usually taken to mean information that will negatively affect the patient's view of his or her future. The degree of bad news is proportional to the distance between the patient's perception of the situation and reality.

Objectives

While bad news can never be made good news, the task of breaking bad news is to close the gap between the patient's perception of the situation and reality. The skill in achieving this lies in controlling the speed at which this transition takes place. Clearly, the larger the distance between the two positions, the more difficult the task and the more skill required.

Process

1. Interview preparation. Adequate time and preparation are essential to avoid psychological scarring for the patient. This can be started at earlier consultations by indicating to the patient any investigations that may confirm clinical suspicions. This can also be a time to determine how much information the patient wants to hear and whether they want a relative or friend with them when any potentially bad news is given.

The doctor should not appear rushed and should have the correct medical information to hand. Reading written reports of investigations leads to less confusion than relying on verbal messages. Privacy is desirable and the patient should be given the opportunity of having a relative present if they wish.

2. Opening the discussion. A brief introduction establishes the names and relationships of all present. The doctor should sit down near to the patient, make eye contact and avoid distracting mannerisms.

3. Clarifying the patient's coping strategy. The patient's interpretation of their illness should be sought by asking about their symptoms, the results of tests so far and what treatment they have had. After the patient's story has been clarified, the patient should be asked whether he/she wishes the doctor to explain further about the illness or the latest results. Patients should not have information forced upon them.

4. Breaking the bad news. If the patient wishes to be told more information, the doctor can proceed to tell them by warning that there is bad news, explaining slowly and checking understanding frequently. Euphemisms should be avoided and it is usually best to use the word cancer at some stage. The doctor should tell the news at the patient's pace and appreciate that they may not remember or understand much of what is said in these circumstances. Simplified anatomical diagrams can help the process.

5. Handling responses. Many patients cry when they hear that they have cancer or that treatment has failed. The doctor should avoid looking embarrassed and should let the patient know that it is normal behaviour to express feelings. Anger is a common response and it is best to let the patient talk while the doctor remains calm and avoids being defensive. Information can take a while to sink in and the patient will be silent for a while. Often this only takes a minute or so and the doctor should resist offering false hope during this time but instead empathize with the patient and allow him/her space to think.

6. Identifying other concerns. Once the news has been told and sunk in, the patient may express particular concerns about treatment or symptoms. These can be addressed at this time or at a later interview if the patient wishes. Quoting inflated success rates for treatment should be avoided as it can lead to bitterness and anger later if they fail.

7. Discussing prognosis. Questions about survival are asked by many patients. It may be better to describe the range of possibilities than to guess at a precise figure as this is usually wrong. Some patients confront the doctor with "Am I going to die ?" and this deserves an honest response in a sensitive way. "The cancer will shorten your life" is one option that allows further exploration if the patient wishes.

8. *Closing the interview.* The doctor should warn the patient that they are leaving shortly and ask the patient if they have any other worries or questions. Re-assurance about continuing support can be offered and plans made for another consultation soon. It may be helpful to point out that most normal people find it difficult to retain all of the information from these discussions and that further opportunities to clarify the situation will be available. A written record of what the patient has been told is important as is communication with other health-care professionals.

Difficult areas

Denial. This can be a useful coping mechanism but may be challenged when it causes significant anguish for the patient or relative and if it stops a patient from dealing with important issues for them and family members.

Collusion with relatives. A conspiracy of silence can lead to a lonely, isolated death if the patient is not given the opportunity of knowing their diagnosis. It is usually appropriate to challenge collusion to spare the patient the anxiety and distress of isolation. This also avoids a complicated bereavement for relatives, who were prevented from being open with the patient by their conspiracy. In general, clinical information should be first discussed with the patient and only with the relatives if the patient has given permission for the doctor to do so. One technique for dealing with a relative not wishing that the patient be told the diagnosis is to explore the reasons behind this and negotiate access to the patient. The doctor can reassure the relative that if the patient does not want to be told then this will be respected. Careful record should be made of any decision to contravene relatives wishes after discussion with colleagues in the team.

This topic is distilled from Bennett M, Alison D. Discussing the diagnosis and prognosis with cancer patients. *Postgraduate Medical Journal,* 1996; **72:** 25–29, with permission from the *Postgraduate Medical Journal.*

Further reading

Doyle D, Hartes G, Macdonald N. *Oxford Textbook of Palliative Medicine,* Oxford Medical Publications, 1993.

Related topic of interest

Palliative care (p. 194)

BREAST CANCER

Background

Incidence

Carcinoma of the breast is the most common cancer in women, accounting for 19% of all new cases of female cancer. In the UK, 26 000 new cases are diagnosed each year and approximately 16 000 women die from the disease. It is estimated that in the UK 1 in 12 women will develop breast cancer. It is a rare cancer in men.

Risk factors

Factors which increase the risk of breast cancer include increasing age, late childbearing, nulliparity, early menarche, late menopause, family history (first degree relative, particularly premenopausal), obesity and ionizing radiation.

Inherited mutations of certain genes confer a familial predisposition to breast cancer. Mutations of the *BRCA1* gene are associated with an increased susceptibility to breast and ovarian cancer. Mutations of the *BRCA2* gene have been linked with early onset breast cancer and male breast cancer, but not with ovarian cancer.

Histology

Infiltrating or invasive ductal carcinoma is the most common cell type, comprising 70–80% of all cases. Lobular carcinoma, comprising approximately 10% of cases, is characterized by a higher incidence of multicentric tumours within the same or opposite breast. Other less common histological types include medullary, colloid, comedo and papillary.

Tumours are graded according to differentiation with grade 1 lesions being well differentiated and grade 3 lesions being poorly differentiated.

Clinical features

Presentation

Most patients present with a breast mass. Less common presentation is with nipple discharge, regional lymphadenopathy (axillary or supraclavicular nodes), or with symptoms of metastatic disease.

Mammographic detection of clinically occult malignancy found on routine mammography is becoming more common (see below).

Investigations

Diagnosis should be confirmed by fine-needle aspiration cytology (FNAC), needle biopsy, incisional or excisional biopsy.

All patients should have bilateral mammography performed prior to any definitive local treatment to detect multicentric tumours or synchronous primaries in the opposite breast.

In patients at high risk of disseminated disease, consideration should be given to performing isotopic bone scan and liver imaging with ultrasound or CT scanning.

Staging

Definitive staging of breast cancer uses the TNM system.

T0   No primary tumour.
T1   Tumour less than 2 cm.
T2   Tumour between 2 and 5 cm.
T3   Primary tumour greater than 5 cm.
T4   Skin involvement.

N0   No lymph nodes.
N1   Mobile axillary nodes.
N2   Fixed axillary nodes.
N3   Internal mammary nodes.

M0   No metastases.
M1   Distant metastases.

Breast cancer is frequently staged as follows.

Stage 0:   *in-situ* breast cancer.
Stage I: small moveable tumour confined to the breast.
Stage II: as stage I, but with spread to the ipsilateral axillary lymph nodes. (Nodes not fixed.)
Stage III: locally advanced tumour possibly attached to chest muscles.
Stage IV: Distant metastasis present.

Management

Surgery

Surgery is the treatment of choice for localized disease. Surgical options include mastectomy (radical or simple) or conservative surgery (e.g. wide local excision) with postoperative radiotherapy. Survival is equivalent with any of these options in appropriately selected patients. Selection of the appropriate therapeutic approach depends on the location and size of the lesion, breast size, appearance on the mammogram, the extent of *in situ* change and patient preference.

An assessment of axillary lymph node disease should be performed in all patients with high-risk disease. This may occur as a secondary procedure following the initial resection of the primary tumour.

In some cases of isolated local recurrence, further surgical resection (sometimes in conjunction with other treatment modalities) can be curative.

Radiotherapy

Following conservative surgery, all patients require radiotherapy to the residual breast tissue. Local radiotherapy may also be indicated following mastectomy in those who are assessed as having a high risk of local recurrence [e.g. deep resection margin involvement, large primary tumours (>4 cm), multiple axillary lymph nodes containing metastatic disease, and widespread lymphovascular tumour permeation].

When a full axillary dissection has been performed, axillary radiotherapy should not be routinely given. However, it should be considered in individual cases when the risk of local recurrence is particularly high (e.g. extensive extracapsular disease). The increased risk of lymphoedema in this situation should be discussed with the patient prior to radiotherapy.

In recurrent breast cancer, radiotherapy has a major role in the palliation of locally recurrent disease and controlling symptoms such as pain due to bony metastasis.

Systemic therapy

Systemic therapy with endocrine treatment or with cytotoxic chemotherapy is of proven value for the treatment of both micrometastatic disease in an adjuvant setting and recurrent/metastatic disease.

The following factors may be considered in selecting treatment:

- Hormone receptor status [oestrogen receptor (ER) status].
- Menopausal status.
- Sites of recurrent disease (e.g. visceral or soft tissue lesions).
- Disease-free interval.
- Response to previous treatment.
- Performance status.

Endocrine therapy

Adjuvant.

(a) Tamoxifen therapy, 20 mg/day, significantly reduces the annual risk of recurrence (by approximately 25%) and of death (17%) in the adjuvant setting. The benefit in patients whose primary tumours are ER negative is approximately half that seen in patient with ER-positive tumours. A reduced incidence of contralateral breast cancer and reduced cardiovascular mortality has also been reported. Tamoxifen, in this schedule is associated with an increased risk of endometrial carcinoma at least twice that of untreated women.

(b) Ovarian ablation has also been shown to significantly reduce the risk of recurrence in premenopausal women in the adjuvant setting. This may be performed by either oophorectomy or radiotherapy-induced menopause.

Metastatic disease. One third of unselected patients with metastatic disease respond to endocrine therapies. The median duration of response to a single endocrine therapy is 1–2 years. The chance of an objective response is significantly higher in patients with ER-positive tumours (50–60%) compared with patients with ER-negative tumours (5–10%).

A higher response rate to endocrine therapy can also be related to several other factors:

(a) The dominant site of disease (highest in women with disease in soft tissue, less in those with bone metastasis and less again in those with visceral metastasis).

(b) An objective response to prior endocrine treatment.

(c) Greater duration of previous disease-free interval.

Therapeutic options include:

(a) Ovarian ablation. In premenopausal women, endogenous ovarian oestrogen production may be stopped by ovarian ablation (surgically or radiotherapy induced) or by the use of luteinizing hormone releasing hormone agonists.

(b) Antioestrogens (e.g. Tamoxifen at a dose of 20 mg/day, which should be continued until documented evidence of disease recurrence).

(c) Progesterones. Semisynthetic progesterones such as medroxy-progesterone acetate and megestrol acetate.

(d) Aromatase inhibitors (e.g. aminoglutethamide). The new aromatase inhibitors appear to have equal efficacy to aminoglutethamide, with fewer side effects.

Chemotherapy

Adjuvant. Combination chemotherapy significantly reduces the annual risk of recurrent breast cancer (~28%) and mortality (~16%) when used in the adjuvant setting. The effect is greater in women less than 50 years of age. Common regimes include CMF (cyclophosphamide/methotrexate/5-FU) and anthracycline containing combination regimens such as FEC (5-FU/epirubucin/cyclophosphamide) which are probably of equal efficacy.

The dose intensity of adjuvant treatment is important as a reduction of dose compromises outcome.

Metastatic disease. In the setting of disseminated breast carcinoma, the aim of conventional chemotherapy is to palliate symptoms and improve quality of life. Combination chemotherapy is generally more effective than single agents, the exception being single agent doxorubicin which is as effective as several standard combination regimes.

Combination chemotherapy regimes include:

- CMF: cyclophosphamide/methotrexate/5-FU.
- AC: Doxorubicin (adriamycin)/cyclophosphamide.

- FAC: 5-FU/doxorubicin/cyclophosphamide.
- FEC: 5-FU/epirubucin /cyclophosphamide.
- MMM: methotrexate/mitomycin C/mitozantrone.

Response rates with combination chemotherapy in previously untreated patients range from 45 to 80%, with a median duration of response of 5–13 months. Response rates for second line therapy are significantly lower. The optimal duration of chemotherapy in this setting is controversial. Newer agents such as the taxanes seem to be at least as effective as these standard regimens.

Prognostic factors

Stage of tumour

Stage I: 84% 5 year survival.
Stage II: 71% 5 year survival.
Stage III: 48% 5 year survival.
Stage IV: 18% 5 year survival.

Histology

Prognosis is also dependent on histological grade, nuclear grade and oestrogen receptor status. Peritumoural lymphatic vessel invasion, tumour microvessel density, proliferative capacity of primary tumour, *c-erb-B2* (HER-2), *c-myc* and *p53* expression by the tumour may also be important.

Screening

In women aged 50 years and over, breast screening by mammography should result in a reduction in breast mortality ranging from 15 to 20%. For women under the age of 50 years, no significant mortality reduction has been demonstrated.

Current issues

Endocrine therapy

Trials are ongoing to assess the optimal duration of tamoxifen therapy in the adjuvant setting

Immunotherapy

The use of a recombinant humanized monoclonal antibody to *c-ERB-B2* (HER-2) is currently being investigated in phase III trials in metastatic breast cancer.

High-dose chemotherapy The use of high-dose chemotherapy with peripheral blood stem cell support has shown promising results in phase II studies, in both the adjuvant and recurrent disease setting. One recent small randomized phase III study reported a survival benefit in women with metastatic disease. However, the results of ongoing randomized phase III trials are currently being awaited.

Further reading

Dixon JM, ed. *ABC of Breast Diseases.* BMJ Publishing Group, 1995.

Related topic of interest

Tamoxifen (p. 250)

CANCER IMAGING – PRINCIPLES

Imaging has a central role in the diagnosis, staging and treatment of cancer. The ability to non-invasively define tumour site, size, extent and dissemination is continuously improving as imaging technology evolves. Diagnostic and therapeutic interventional techniques further expand the role of radiologists. The contribution of imaging to certain cancer screening programmes is also well established.

Uses of imaging in cancer medicine

Diagnosis

Radiological investigation forms part of the initial assessment of almost all patients with cancer. Although many tumours produce a characteristic radiological appearance, histology is required to make an accurate diagnosis. For an increasing number of patients, guided biopsy under local anaesthesia performed by a radiologist can provide an adequate specimen for histological or cytological diagnosis and may obviate the need for more invasive surgical intervention.

Staging

The cornerstone of staging lies in precise definition of the anatomical extent of disease. This is now achieved non-invasively with cross-sectional imaging techniques. CT is the standard imaging tool for the evaluation of chest and abdomino-pelvic malignancies. The uses of MRI are ever increasing.

Response

Radiological investigation plays a key role in defining the response to treatment in addition to other markers (clinical status, tumour markers). CT is used as a reproducible technique, accurately measuring changes in tumour dimensions. Conventional examinations such as chest radiography are also used to monitor disease response when appropriate.

Follow-up

When detection of asymptomatic relapse has been shown to affect clinical outcome (e.g. testicular tumours) further use of radiology for surveillance is justified. However, in other cancers (e.g. ovarian carcinoma) routine follow-up imaging has not been formally demonstrated to affect prognosis.

Screening

The use of screening mammography to detect breast cancer is now well established in the UK. The use of other radiological screening examinations has not been widely accepted (e.g. CXR to assess people at high risk of lung cancers, transvaginal ultrasound for ovarian cancer and transrectal ultrasound for prostate cancer).

Imaging techniques

In addition to routine conventional radiography the full range of imaging techniques are used in cancer medicine. The cross-sectional techniques of CT and magnetic resonance imaging (MRI) obviously have a dominant role.

CT

Data are acquired using a rotating X-ray tube housed in a fixed gantry with computed reconstruction of axial cross-sectional images, based solely on the X-ray attenuation of the tissues. Image quality has improved and scan times dramatically shortened by technological advances such as helical (spiral) CT. Section thickness of between 1 and 10 mm are used depending upon the application. Oral contrast medium may be administered to outline the GI tract. This can demonstrate intra-luminal pathology or bowel obstruction and avoid misinterpretation of bowel loops as mass lesions. Intravenous contrast medium is used to delineate vascular structures and to demonstrate tumour enhancement, thus increasing lesion detection, particularly in the liver.

MRI

The principle of nuclear magnetic resonance has been exploited to develop a clinical imaging tool that produces images of high soft-tissue contrast in any cross-sectional plane. These advantages mean that MRI is now the gold standard for imaging neurospinal, head and neck and musculoskeletal tumours. Dangers from exposure to a strong magnetic field within which the image is acquired may preclude some patients from being examined (e.g. those with a cardiac pacemaker).

Ultrasound

The reflection of high-frequency sound waves at soft tissue interfaces generates the ultrasound image. Ultrasound, requiring no ionizing radiation, is safe, widely available and inexpensive. Apart from detecting metastases in solid visceral abdominal organs, specialist applications such as duplex and doppler ultrasound are used to assess tumour blood flow. This can contribute to the characterization of some neoplastic masses. Ultrasound is also used for real-time guidance of biopsy and therapeutic interventional procedures.

Nuclear medicine

Radioisotope-labelled pharmaceuticals are administered intravenously, and their distribution measured by γ-camera detection of emitted photons. Bone scintigraphy remains the principal investigation for detection of skeletal metastases.

Current issues

PET scanning

Positron emission tomography uses high-energy photons emitted by short-lived isotopes produced by a cyclotron. It has the potential to differentiate malignant from benign pathologies, but its availability remains limited.

Further reading

Bragg DG, Rubin P, Youker JE, eds. *Oncologic Imaging*, Oxford: Pergamon Press, Chapters 1, 2.

Carr DT. Is staging of cancer of value? *Cancer,* 1983; **51:** 2503–5.

The Use of Computed Tomography in the Initial Investigation of Common Malignancies. Council, Royal College of Radiologists, 1994.

CELL CYCLE

The cell cycle refers to the process of cell division. In normal tissues this process is tightly controlled by the activity of a number of key cellular proteins. A loss of cell cycle control may lead to an inappropriate proliferation of cells and ultimately, to tumour formation.

Cell cycle phases

The cell cycle is divided into four phases:

1. *Mitosis (M)*. The phase during which the cell under goes division into two daughter cells.

2. *Gap 1 (G1)*. The phase between M and S.

3. *Synthesis (S)*. The phase during which chromosome replication occurs.

4. *Gap 2 (G2)*. The phase between S and M.

When cells stop actively dividing they leave the cell cycle (usually at G1) and enter a resting phase generally known as G0.

Checkpoint control

Transition from one phase of the cell cycle to the next is tightly controlled at specific points known as checkpoints. The major checkpoints control transition from G1 to S and G2 to M. Transition through the cell cycle checkpoints is regulated by protein complexes consisting of cyclins, cyclin-dependent kinases and their inhibitors.

Cdk. The cyclin-dependent kinases are a family of enzymes (Cdk2, Cdk4, Cdk6, Cdc2, etc.) that phosphorylate substrate proteins (such as Rb) and control the transition from one phase of the cell cycle to the next. Specific checkpoints are associated with the activity of certain Cdks, for example the G1–S checkpoint is controlled by Cdk4 and Cdk6.

Cyclin. The cyclins are regulatory proteins that bind to, and thus control, the activity of the Cdks. A number of cyclins have been identified (cyclins A, B, C, D, E and

G). They show a degree of specificity as to how Cdk is bound, for example cyclin D binds to Cdk4 and Cdk6. Although the levels of the Cdks are relatively constant throughout the cell cycle, the levels of cyclins rise and fall at specific points, thus activating their partner Cdks in a cycle-specific manner.

CKI. The cyclin-dependent kinase inhibitors are a group of proteins that negatively control the activity of the Cdk–cyclin complexes. The CKIs inhibit the activity of the Cdks by binding to the Cdk–cyclin complex or directly to the Cdk preventing the binding of the partner cyclin. These two families of CKI have various members, usually named by their molecular weight in kd, for example p16, p21, p27.

G1–S checkpoint

Transition through the G1–S checkpoint commits a cell to undergo division. The control of the G1–S checkpoint exemplifies the integration of the various components of the cell cycle machinery.

G1–S checkpoint transition is brought about by phosphorylation of the retinoblastoma protein (pRb). This ubiquitous protein is phosphorylated by a cyclin-D-dependent Cdk. This phosphorylation releases factors that lead to the transcription of genes required for DNA synthesis, such as DNA polymerases, enabling the cell to enter the S phase. G1–S transition is inhibited through the action of the CKIs particularly p21. p21 binds directly to Cdks inhibiting activation by cyclin D. This prevents phosphorylation of the Rb protein and cell cycle progression is inhibited.

Cell cycle and cancer

Abnormalities in the cell cycle of cancer cells may lead to abnormal proliferation and/or a failure to respond appropriately to DNA damage (repair or apoptosis).

Abnormal proliferation

Aberrant cell proliferation may result from a variety of abnormalities in cell cycle machinery.

Proteins that promote cell cycle progression, such as the cyclins, are frequently overexpressed in neoplastic cells.

- Cyclin D overexpression is described in B-cell lymphomas (as a result of the 11:14 translocation), breast, oesophagus and bladder cancer.

Proteins that normally inhibit cell cycle progression are frequently inactivated in cancer cells (i.e. act as tumour-suppressor genes).

- CKI inactivation has been identified in glioblastomas, bladder carcinomas, malignant mesotheliomas, familial melanoma and leukaemias.
- pRb inactivation occurs in all retinoblastomas and is seen in both non-small cell and small cell carcinoma of the lung and bladder and in pancreatic carcinomas.

DNA damage

In a normal cell DNA damage is either repaired or leads to death of the cell by apoptosis. Both of these processes require cell cycle arrest.

DNA damage leads to cell cycle arrest in a p53-dependent manner. p53 is a transcriptional activator for p21, that is it binds to the p21 gene sequence and increases its transcription, which in turn leads to increased levels of the protein. An increase in p53 thus leads to an increase in p21, which in turn inhibits the activity of the cyclin D dependent Cdks and prevents phosphorylation of pRb, arresting the cell at the G1–S checkpoint.

Abnormalities in this DNA damage response mechanism, for example p53 mutations, therefore allow both escape from apoptosis and accumulation of further mutations.

Chemotherapy

Certain chemotherapy drugs act in a cell cycle specific manner, that is their action predominates in one specific phase of the cell cycle.

S phase specific. Drugs that specifically inhibit DNA synthesis are S phase specific, for example antimetabolites such as methotrexate and cytarabine.

M phase specific. Drugs that inhibit the formation of the mitotic spindle and chromosome segregation are M phase specific, for example vincristine and Taxol.

Many chemotherapy combinations attempt to combine drugs which act at different phases of the cell cycle.

Future directions
The cell cycle and its abnormalities in malignant cells is a major focus of cancer research. Drugs targeted against protein components of the cell cycle are being developed.

Further reading

Fisler RP. CDKs and cyclins in transition(s). *Science*, 1996; **274:** 1672–7.
Sherr CJ. Cancer cell cycles. *Science,* 1996; **274:** 1672–77.

Related topics of interest

Apoptosis (p. 4)
Cervical cancer (p. 44)
Head and neck cancer (p. 105)
Molecular biology of cancer (p. 151)

CERVICAL CANCER

Background

Incidence

Cancer of the cervix is the second most common female cancer worldwide. In the UK approximately 5000 cases of invasive carcinoma and more than 20 000 cases of carcinoma *in situ* are diagnosed each year.

Risk factors

Early age of sexual activity, multiple partners, parity and chronic inflammation are associated with an increased risk. The incidence is increased in lower social classes, smokers and women with a history of cervical dysplasia. The relationship to oral contraceptive use is not yet clear. Carcinoma of the cervix is extremely rare in nuns.

Aetiology

Sexual activity is an important factor in the development of carcinoma of the cervix and a causative role for sexually transmitted infectious agents has been proposed, [human papilloma viruses (HPV) types 16 and 18]. The HPV proteins E6 and E7 bind and inactivate p53 and pRb respectively, dysregulating cell cycle control.

Histology

Carcinoma of the cervix develops at the squamocolumnar junction. Pre-invasive lesions of the cervix, cervical intraepithelial neoplasia (CIN), are graded according to the degree of cytological abnormality, CIN 1 to 3. Carcinoma *in situ* (CIN 3) is a pre-invasive malignancy although it may take many years to become invasive. Not all CIN 1 and 2 lesions progress to invasive carcinoma.

Approximately 85% of invasive lesions are squamous cell carcinomas, 5–10% are adenocarcinomas. Primary sarcoma, lymphoma or adenoacanthomas of the cervix are also seen.

Clinical features

Presentation

Carcinoma *in situ* is asymptomatic and may be detected on a routine Papanicolaou smear. Most patients with carcinoma *in situ* have an area of redness on the portio vaginalis of the cervix which resembles chronic cervicitis. Invasive cancers usually present with vaginal bleeding or discharge, especially post-coital. Pain may be a presenting feature including abdominal pain, low back pain and dyspareunia. Urinary and rectal symptoms may occur in locally extensive disease.

Investigations

Positive cervical cytology should be followed up with colposcopy and biopsy. Accurate staging is achieved with a combination of clinical (including an examination under anaesthesia) and radiological examination. Sigmoidoscopy and intravenous urography, previously performed in all cases, are increasingly being replaced with CT.

Staging

The most commonly used staging system is that of the International Federation of Gynaecology and Obstetrics (FIGO).

Stage 0:   carcinoma *in situ*.
Stage 1:   disease confined to cervix.
    1a: micro-invasive carcinoma.
    1b: occult and clinical invasive carcinoma.
Stage 2:   disease beyond cervix but not to the pelvic wall.
    2a: no parametrial involvement evident.
    2b: parametrial involvement.
Stage 3:   extension to pelvic side wall and/or lower third of vagina.
    3a: no extension to pelvic side wall.
    3b: extension to pelvic side wall and/or hydronephrosis or non-functioning kidney.
Stage 4:   carcinoma beyond true pelvis or involving mucosa of bladder or rectum.
    4a: spread to local organs.
    4b: spread to distant organs.

Management

Surgery

Carcinoma in situ can usually be cured with a therapeutic cone biopsy. Local ablation using laser surgery, cryotherapy or electrocoagulation can be used in selected cases. A total hysterectomy may be performed if future child-bearing is not an issue.

Invasive carcinoma of the cervix stages 1 and 2a may be treated with either surgery or radiotherapy. More advanced disease is usually managed with radiotherapy although in selected cases a pelvic exenteration may be performed.

Surgery involves a radical (Wertheim's) hysterectomy with removal of a 2–3 cm cuff of vagina, all supporting tissues within the true pelvis in addition to a complete pelvic lymph node dissection. This operation should ideally be performed by a surgeon specializing in oncological gynaecology.

Radiotherapy

Radiotherapy is widely used in carcinoma of the cervix especially for patients presenting with more advanced disease. In most cases both intracavitary and external sources are used.

Intracavitary treatment involves the placement of radioactive sources in the uterus and in the lateral vaginal fornices. This delivers a high dose to the uterus, cervix and upper vagina and a lesser dose to the paracervical and parametrial tissues.

External irradiation to the whole pelvis, with or without a parametrial boost, is usually used in combination with intracavitary treatment. Intracavitary treatment is considered to be more important in early disease and external irradiation more important in later stages.

Chemotherapy

Chemotherapy has an increasing role in advanced or recurrent disease. The response rates are usually higher when chemotherapy is used as the primary treatment. This may be due to the altered blood supply after surgery or radiotherapy or it may be that recurrent or persistent cancer cells are more resistant.

Responses have been seen with several agents, with cisplatin being the most active, having a single agent response rate of 20–30%. Chemotherapy has not, however, been associated with a definite survival advantage to date. Cisplatin-based regimes are most frequently used. The combination of bleomycin, ifosfamide and cisplatin (BIP) is often used in advanced disease, with response rates of approximately 50–60%.

The efficiency of adjuvant and neoadjuvant chemotherapy is unproven.

Prognostic factors

Stage of tumour

Stage 1: 80–90% 5 year survival.
Stage 2: 60% 5 year survival.
Stage 3: 30% 5 year survival.
Stage 4: <10% 5 year survival.

Screening

The marked difference in survival between the different stages underlies the importance of detecting the disease early. Screening by regular cervical smear is now widespread in the Western world and has contributed to a fall in the development of invasive disease and the overall death rate.

The screening programme in the UK aims to screen all women aged between 20 and 64 every 5 years. Screening every 3 years further reduces the incidence of invasive carcinoma. A programme which screens approximately 80% of women could lead to a mortality reduction of 65–70%.

Current issues

Adjuvant therapy

The role of adjuvant chemotherapy following surgery or radiotherapy in high-risk patients is being evaluated. Neoadjuvant chemotherapy appears promising in patients presenting with locally advanced disease although randomized controlled trials are needed to assess this.

Vaccination

Vaccination strategies directed against the viral oncoproteins E6 and E7 of the HPV-16 and -18 are being developed to prevent the development of cervical carcinoma.

Screening

PCR can detect HPV in cervical smears and positive results correlate with cervical cancer. The role of this technique in screening is being evaluated.

Related topic of interest

Cell cycle (p. 40)

CHEMOTHERAPY – (a) GENERAL PRINCIPLES

The mainstay of systemic therapy for cancer is chemotherapy although hormonal and biological treatments can play an important role. Chemotherapy for solid tumours has only been developed since the 1940s. With the introduction of newer cytotoxic drugs the ability to affect the natural progression of a tumour has increased and in several malignancies, cure is a real possibility.

Indications

The indications for the use of chemotherapy are varied but they should be clearly defined at the start of treatment. Chemotherapy treatment can be used in the following roles.

Neoadjuvant
Primary treatment of a tumour before definitive surgical intervention. The aims of this are to make the tumour smaller, rendering it operable or to allow less radical surgery, while at the same time treating micrometastases. This approach is established for osteosarcoma and is being tested in clinical trials for other tumour malignancies such as breast cancer.

Adjuvant
The use of chemotherapy following surgery that has achieved complete macroscopic clearance. Chemotherapy in this setting treats the microscopic metastases which could lead to relapse (e.g. breast cancer and colorectal cancer).

Palliative
This is treatment to alleviate symptoms and in some cases prolong life in patients who cannot be cured. Chemotherapy given in the palliative setting has to be a carefully balanced decision so that the patients quality of life is not made worse by the treatment. It may be justified to give second or third line chemotherapy if the disease remains chemosensitive (e.g. breast cancer, ovarian cancer, small cell lung cancer).

Curative
In some malignancies there is still a real chance of a cure even if there is metastatic disease at presentation (e.g. germ cell tumours, Hodgkin's disease, non-Hodgkin's lymphoma and many childhood cancers). This justifies the use of more intensive treatment associated with greater toxicity.

Prophylactic	Hormonal treatments may be given before overt malignancy appears. For instance tamoxifen may be used for *in situ* breast cancer before invasive carcinoma is recognized.

Chemotherapy principles

Combination	Cytotoxic chemotherapy is most commonly given as a combination of different drugs. This is because different classes of drugs have different actions and may work synergistically. Using this approach there is also less chance of drug-resistant malignant cells emerging. Ideally drugs with different toxicities are combined. Single-agent chemotherapy may be appropriate, especially in the palliative setting.
Scheduling	Most chemotherapy is given cyclically to allow normal cells to recover from the toxicity of treatment. The cells usually affected at standard doses are haematopoietic stem cells and the lining of the GI tract, producing myelosuppression and mucositis. Giving the treatment every 3–4 weeks allows these cells to recover. Theoretically any cycle of chemotherapy will only kill a proportion of the tumour cells. Therefore repeated cycles are required to get tumour clearance. However, there is no justification for giving endless cycles of chemotherapy as resistance will emerge.
Dose	*Conventional.* These are doses of drugs known to be effective against the particular malignancy which in the majority of patients do not cause severe side effects. Many of these treatments can be given in an outpatient setting. *High dose.* These are much higher doses of the drugs than standard treatments and therefore the toxicity is much greater. In most cases these patients require some form of bone marrow support (i.e. growth factors, haematopoietic stem cells or bone marrow infusion). This toxicity of this treatment is justified only when long-term survival or cure are possible.

Maintenance	The use of prolonged chemotherapy to maintain a remission has little advantage in solid tumours as resistant clones soon develop. In childhood leukaemia however, the use of 18 months maintenance chemotherapy following the induction of a complete remission is of benefit.

Other treatments

Hormonal	Many cancers appear to be hormone sensitive (e.g. breast and prostate cancers). If the hormone 'drive' is removed by ovarian ablation or orchidectomy the tumours regress. Hormonal drug therapy, such as tamoxifen, has evolved in response to these observations.
Biological	Biological agents such as cytokines may have direct anti-tumour activity or interact with host mechanisms to potentiate natural anti-tumour activity. Other therapies include monoclonal antibodies, vaccinations and gene therapy approaches.

Modes of administration

Orally	Oral chemotherapy has the advantage of reducing hospital visits. However, only a minority of drugs such as cyclophosphamide, etoposide, chlorambucil and tamoxifen are available orally.
Systemically	Most chemotherapy is given intravenously as bolus injection or short infusion. Some chemotherapy may be given as a continuous infusion via a tunnelled line.
Regionally	*1. Intravesical.* Chemotherapy is routinely given intravesically in the management of superficial bladder cancer. This has the advantage of producing high doses at the site of the tumour with negligible systemic absorption and hence minimal systemic toxicity. *2. Intraperitoneal.* Chemotherapy may be administered directly into the peritoneal cavity in the context of

tumours which spread trans-coelomically (e.g. ovarian cancer).

3. Intra-arterial. Any tumour that has a well-defined blood supply is potentially suitable for intra-arterial chemotherapy (e.g. hepatic artery infusion for liver metastases). This allows higher doses to be delivered to the involved site and reduces systemic toxicity.

Related topics of interest

CHEMOTHERAPY – (b) COMBINATION

Single agent chemotherapy is rarely curative and therefore the majority of chemotherapy is given as a combination of different agents. The rationale for combination chemotherapy is that the addition of cytotoxic drugs (with significant response rates when used alone) can produce improved response and survival rates.

The main aims for the use of combination chemotherapy regimens are:

- Maximization of tumour kill.
- Minimization of toxicity to non-tumour cells.
- Minimization of the development of resistance.

Maximizing tumour kill

Malignant tumours are comprised of heterogeneous populations of cells which have variable sensitivities to different chemotherapy agents. The combination of a number of drugs aims to overcome the resistance of any individual population to a single agent. Cells tend to show cross-resistance to drugs with the same mode of cytotoxicity. Therefore drugs with different modes of action are frequently combined to increase the extent of tumour cell killing. For example, drugs such as the anti-metobolites may be combined with alkylating agents. This greater reduction in tumour cell number reduces the chance of resistant clones developing. For most cancer cells, a relationship exists between dose of chemotherapy and killing. Ideally each drug used in combination is given at a dose similar to the maximally tolerated dose when used as a single agent.

To further maximize tumour cell killing, repeated cycles of chemotherapy are used. A cell kill of 99% per cycle represents only a 2 log reduction i.e. from 10^9 (clinically detectable) to 10^7 cells. Repeated cycles, each with a 2 log reduction in cell number, are therefore essential to reduce the residual number of tumour cells below that required to achieve a cure.

Minimizing toxicity

All chemotherapy agents are toxic to normal cells Different agents may have different toxicity profiles. Combining effective drugs with non-overlapping toxicity allows anti-tumour effect to be maximized without causing severe toxicity to normal cells, e.g. the combination of nephrotoxic cisplatin with haematologically toxic alkylating agents in the management of ovarian cancer. The combination of two or more drugs with similar ad verse effects may lead to severe toxicity. By minimizing additive toxicities the dose of each agent can be increased leading to an increase in overall dose intensity.

The administration of chemotherapy at defined intervals allows recovery of normal tissues prior to the administration of further chemotherapy. The interval between cycles may be different for different regimes reflecting the recovery time required, e.g. the myelosuppression induced by carboplatin is longer than most drugs and therefore a 4-week interval is used rather than the standard 3 weeks. These intervals are a balance between allowing normal cells to recover and maximizing 'toxicity' to the tumour cell.

Minimizing drug resistance Drug resistance is either a primary characteristic of the initial malignant clone or can be acquired through the multiple genetic events which occur in tumour progression. The combination of several drugs increases the probability of killing the initial population. With reduced numbers of malignant cells, the chance of a resistant clone developing is reduced.

Design of combination chemotherapy regimes

Important factors in designing clinically useful combination chemotherapy regimes include:

- Use of cytotoxic drugs restricted to those with significant single agent activity.
- Use of cytotoxic drugs with non-overlapping toxicities.
- Use of cytotoxic drugs at their optimal dose intensity, i.e. dose and frequency.
- Use of cytotoxic drugs to which there are different modes of resistance.

Although based on rational principles, the development of complex combination chemotherapy regimes is often empirical, with the optimum combination of cytotoxics, their individual doses and scheduling arrived at by continuous re-evaluation. New combinations are constantly being devised and developed and should be tested within the context of a clinical trial.

Examples of combination chemotherapy regimes

Two examples of combination chemotherapy are the CHOP and BEP regimes. These two regimes are also important in that they are the highly effective and potentially curative treatments for lymphomas and germ cell tumours, respectively.

CHOP   C   Cyclophosphamide – 750 mg/m^2 as bolus injection
H   Hydroxy-daunorubicin* – 50 mg/m^2 as bolus injection
O   Vincristine (Oncovin®) – 2 mg bolus IV injection
P   Prednisolone – 100 mg per day for 5 days, orally
* Ilydroxy-daunorubicin – Doxorubicin – Adriamycin

- This is repeated every 3 weeks, with nadir blood counts often assessed 10–14 days after initial treatment to ensure appropriate doses are used.
- The bolus injections allow out-patient administration.
- At each cycle an assessment must be made of both the toxicity and response to previous cycles.
- Prior to administration of the drugs, a full blood count is required to confirm haematological recovery.
- Anti-emetics are required prior to administration of chemotherapy.
- Allopurinol is prescribed with initial cycles to prevent accumulation of uric acid following rapid tumour cell lysis.

BEP

B Bleomycin – 30 IU as bolus injection days 2, 9 and 16.

E Etoposide – 120 mg/m^2 days 1–3, IV infusion in 500 ml of normal saline

P Cisplatin – 20 mg/m^2 days 1–5, IV infusion in 500 ml of normal saline with hydration.

- This is repeated every 3 weeks, generally to a maximum of six cycles.
- BEP is in-patient treatment as cisplatin requires aggressive IV hydration to avoid nephrotoxicity except for the day 9 and 16 bolus injections of bleomycin which can be administered in outpatients.
- At each cycle an assessment must be made of both the toxicity and response to previous cycles.
- Prior to administration of the drugs, a full blood count is required to confirm haematological recovery.
- Renal function must be assessed prior to each cycle of cisplatin.
- Anti-emetics are required prior to administration of chemotherapy.
- Allopurinol is prescribed with initial cycles to prevent accumulation of uric acid following rapid tumour cell lysis.
- The cumulative pulmonary toxicity of bleomycin may require this agent to be omitted in the later cycles.

Related topics of interest

CHEMOTHERAPY – (c) HIGH DOSE

High-dose chemotherapy generally refers to the use of chemotherapy agents at doses which require bone-marrow support. This was previously achieved by bone-marrow transplantation although peripheral haematopoietic progenitors (stem cells) are now more commonly used. High-dose chemotherapy has been used with some success in several haematological malignancies. Standard doses of chemotherapy rarely produce durable remissions in most solid tumours and therefore the role of high-dose chemotherapy remains under evaluation.

Rationale

Standard chemotherapy fails for many reasons. These include:

- The presence of chemo-resistant tumour cells.
- The persistence of chemosensitive tumour cells due to inadequate treatment.
- The acquisition of drug resistance.

Many cytotoxic agents demonstrate a dose–response effect [i.e. increasing the dose increases the fractional cell kill (the percentage of tumour cells killed)]. Higher doses should therefore prevent the persistence of chemosensitive tumour cells. Higher doses may also be capable of overcoming resistance mechanisms.

However, tumours which are totally refractory to standard doses of chemotherapy are unlikely to respond to high-dose treatment. Most patients are therefore treated with an introductory phase of chemotherapy and proceed to higher doses only if the tumour responds. Induction therapy may also reduce the volume of tumour present to a size that can be eradicated by high-dose consolidation.

Progenitor cells

Stem cells can now be collected by leukaphersis of peripheral blood. The early progenitor cells can be recognized by a cell-surface antigen 'CD34'. These cells, predominantly resident in the bone marrow, are mobilized into the peripheral circulation by the administration of recombinant colony-stimulating factors (e.g. G-CSF). This is usually preceded by a priming dose of a myelosuppressive agent such as cyclophosphamide. This increases the numbers of circulating early progenitor cells 10- to 100-fold in 10–14 days. Sufficient numbers are normally collected with two to three leukaphareses.

The principal advantages of peripheral blood stem cell rescue compared with bone-marrow transplantation include the rapidity of the engraftment, the ability to give multiple cycles of chemotherapy, shorter inpatient stay, less tumour contamination of the harvest and reduced costs. The rapidity of the engraftment is thought to be due to the reinfusion of larger numbers of more mature peripheral progenitors.

Treatment

The choice of high-dose chemotherapy regime is determined by the tumour type and treatments previously given. Drug combinations are chosen to avoid overlapping toxicity.

Patients have to be relatively fit before embarking on their treatment. The age of the patient is not an absolute exclusion criteria but poor performance status does preclude this approach.

Prior to high-dose therapy a wide range of investigations are performed which include an assessment of cardiopulmonary function. CMV, HIV, hepatitis B and hepatitis C status are assessed. HLA typing may be performed to enable donor-matched platelets to be given. Sperm samples should be stored particularly for males with potentially curative cancers.

On completion of the stem cell harvest, the chemotherapy is given. The stem cells are reinfused 24–48 hours after the chemotherapy is complete to allow complete drug clearance.

A period of profound neutropenia will follow the chemotherapy and therefore hospitalization is required. The time to engraftment of the stem cells and marrow reconstitution (i.e. the return of acceptable blood counts), takes between 10 and 14 days.

Indications

A role for high-dose chemotherapy is established in the treatment of high-grade non-Hodgkin's lymphoma, Hodgkin's disease, acute and chronic leukaemia and multiple myeloma. In these malignancies high-dose chemotherapy with peripheral stem cell rescue may increase the cure rate significantly.

Its use is still being evaluated but has not been fully substantiated in adjuvant and metastatic breast carcinoma, non-seminomatous germ cell tumours, epithelial ovarian cancer, glioma, sarcoma, small cell lung cancer and low-grade non-Hodgkin's lymphoma.

Toxicity
Despite stem cell support and modern antibiotics, high-dose chemotherapy in specialist centres is still associated with a significant mortality of 1–2%.

With support of the haematological toxicity, pulmonary, CNS and cardiac toxicities become the dose-limiting factors. Other toxicities include severe nausea and vomiting, mucositis, diarrhoea, alopecia, peripheral neuropathies, encephalopathy and sterility.

The long-term complications of high-dose chemotherapy, such as secondary malignancies are not clear. Loss of fertility is normal following these doses of chemotherapy.

Current issues

- The ability of high-dose treatments to improve the survival and cure rate for many solid tumours (e.g. breast carcinoma, teratomas and sarcomas).
- The role of high-dose chemotherapy as adjuvant therapy in high-risk breast cancer.

Further reading

Johnson PWM, Pinkerton R. In: Peckham M, Pinedo H, Veroneri U, eds. *Oxford Textbook of Oncology.* Oxford University Press, 1995; 602–17.

Related topics of interest

Chemotherapy – (a) general principles (p. 48)
Chemotherapy – (b) combination (p. 52)
Chemotherapy – (d) complications (p. 58)
Myelosuppresion (p. 163)

CHEMOTHERAPY – (d) COMPLICATIONS

Chemotherapeutic drugs are toxic agents. Doses at which a therapeutic effect is seen are invariably associated with toxicity. Certain toxicities are drug specific, others reflect the cytoxicity of the drugs on dividing cell populations.

The toxicity associated with chemotherapy drugs must be considered against the potential benefit. Palliative chemotherapy for patients with advanced disease should generally be well tolerated. High-dose chemotherapy is associated with considerable life-threatening toxicity, but this can be justified in situations where cure is possible.

The complications of chemotherapy can be considered as immediate or late. Immediate toxicity is of particular importance in patients receiving chemotherapy for palliative intent. Late complications are most important in the adjuvant setting and in those treatments aimed at being curative.

Immediate complications

Nausea/vomiting

Most cytotoxic drugs can cause a degree of nausea and vomiting, which can normally be controlled to a tolerable level. The nausea arises from a combination of direct stimulation of the vomiting centre, peripheral stimulation and anticipatory causes.

Myelosuppression

Chemotherapy causes bone marrow suppression by killing haematopoetic progenitor cells. This leads to a leucopenia and thrombocytopenia, generally after 10–14 days. The lowest point of this drop is known as the nadir. As progenitors recover the peripheral counts return.

A neutrophil count greater than $1 \times 10^9/l$ is rarely associated with a clinical infection. However, the risk of infection with a count less than $0.5 \times 10^9/l$ is significant.

Haemopoietic recovery occurs after 3–4 weeks, enabling further cycles of chemotherapy to be given.

Gastrointestinal

Gastrointestinal side effects are common with most cytotoxic drugs. Oral mucositis may reflect more general damage to the whole gastrointestinal epithelium, a rapidly dividing cell population susceptible to cytotoxic chemotherapy.

Diarrhoea and constipation occur frequently. Rarely, a paralytic ileus can occur with the vinca alkaloids.

Alopecia

Alopecia results from the effects of the cytotoxic drugs on the rapidly dividing cell population at the hair follicle. The effect is reversible with hair returning when chemotherapy is discontinued. In some cases alopecia can be controlled by the use of a cold cap, which reduces the blood flow to the scalp.

Although alopecia has no inherent medical risk, it is a highly significant toxicity because of its effects on the psychological well-being.

Neurological

Peripheral neuropathies. These occur with the platinum drugs, particularly cisplatin, taxanes and vinca alkaloids. The neuropathy, principally affecting sensory nerves, may recover partially over a period of months, but patients are usually left with a residual deficit.

Autonomic neuropathy. The same pathogenic process that affects peripheral nerves may also lead to autonomic dysfunction.

Central neurological toxicity. Although rare, certain drugs are associated with an idiosyncratic toxicity to the CNS, for example ifosfamide-induced encephalopathy and 5-FU-induced cerebellar toxicity.

Ototoxicity

Cochlear damage rather than auditory nerve damage is believed to be responsible for the high-tone hearing loss associated with cisplatin. The effect is permanent. Pre-existing high-tone hearing damage precludes the use of cisplatin.

Genitourinary

Nephrotoxicity. This occurs with platinum agents, principally cisplatin. The renal excretion of many cytotoxics means that adequate renal function is required to reduce overall toxicity.

Bladder toxicity. Cyclophosphamide and ifosfamide cause haemorrhagic cystitis in a dose-dependent manner.

Cardiac

Doxorubicin is associated with acute cardiac toxicity (arrhythmias). High-dose cyclophosphamide is associated with acute cardiac necrosis. 5-FU may cause coronary artery spasm and therefore induce cardiac ischaemia.

Hepatic	Many drugs cause a transient rise of liver enzymes which return to normal. Rarely, fulminant hepatic failure can occur.
Extravasation	Some cytotoxic drugs are highly vesicant and cause tissue damage on extravasation.
Skin toxicity	*1. Palmar plantar erythema.* Erythema of the palms of the hands and soles of the feet is frequently seen with 5-FU. The cause is unknown.
	2. Photosensitivity. Some drugs such as 5-FU cause photosensitivity and patients should be advised regarding the use of high-factor sun blocks.
	3. Pigmentation. Bleomycin leads to skin and nail pigmentation. It occurs in combination with pulmonary fibrosis and a common pathogenic process is thought to be responsible.
Others	*1. General myalgia and arthralgia.* These are seen with the use of paclitaxel and are usually well controlled with non-steroidal analgesia.
	2. Allergic reactions. Both paclitaxel and docetaxel are associated with frequent hypersensitivity reactions on administration.
	3. Lethargy. General malaise and fatigue are common and frequently debilitating. Their aetiology is unknown but it is probably multi-factorial in origin.

Long-term complications

Second malignancies	Some but not all chemotherapy drugs cause sub-lethal DNA damage which may eventually lead to the genetic changes required to induce a second malignancy. The most carcinogenic of anti-cancer drugs are alkylating agents and procarbazine. With long-term survivors following either curative or adjuvant therapy, the frequency of these events is expected to increase. High-dose chemotherapy is also likely to be associated with an increased risk of second malignancies.

Fertility	Most chemotherapy drugs are associated with a reduction in fertility. Some drugs render patients infertile at standard doses; most patients who have high-dose treatments become infertile. Counselling of patients prior to treatment is required.
	Male patients receiving chemotherapy likely to cause infertility should be considered for sperm storage. Whether all patients or only those likely to survive long-term should be offered this service, is an unresolved ethical issue.
	For female patients, it is possible to store fertilized ova, and cryopreservation of sections of ovary may be routine in the near future.
Pulmonary	Long-term pulmonary damage may result from fibrosis induced by drugs such as bleomycin and busulphan. High-dose or prolonged administration of most alkylating agents is associated with pulmonary fibrosis or pneumonitis.
Cardiac	In addition to the acute conduction defects induced by doxorubicin, cardiac fibrosis may also occur. This effect is predictable and dose-dependent. Younger patients are more susceptible to these effects.
Pyschological	The acute toxicities of chemotherapy may lead to a more prolonged effect on the patient's psychology, adversely affecting the patients quality of life.

Conclusion

As the use of chemotherapy is extended and given to more patients in whom long-term survival is expected, long-term toxicities may become more frequent and clinically more significant.

Related topics of interest

CHROMOSOMAL ABNORMALITIES

Genetic changes are central to the pathogenesis of cancer. These changes can be due to very localized abnormalities such as point mutations of individual genes or due to more gross changes at the chromosomal level, for example deletions and translocations. These changes lead to aberrant expression of tumour-suppressor genes or oncogenes.

The cause of chromosomal abnormalities is poorly understood. There is evidence that abnormal recombination of chromosomes during cell division occurs more often at transcriptionally active sites and the recombination sites of the immunoglobulin gene region.

Most recombinations will be deleterious and lead to cell death. However, cells with recombinations that produce a growth advantage clonally expand.

Mechanisms

Deletion

Loss of chromosomal fragments that code tumour-suppressor genes often predisposes to cancer. Loss of one of two alleles (termed loss of heterozygosity) by chromosomal deletion and subsequent mutation in the single remaining allele leads to loss of protein function and the development of malignancy. Detection of regions with frequent loss of heterozygosity by karyotype analysis is used in research to try and identify tumour-suppressor genes.

Amplification

Duplication of certain regions of the chromosome with overexpression of oncogenes may also be associated with tumour formation, for example amplification of the *myc* gene leading to overexpression of myc protein, a cell-cycle related protein. In neuroblastoma, the number of copies of the *myc* gene is related to prognosis.

Translocations

The translocation of chromosomal fragments either places the coding region of one gene under the control of another's control elements or juxtaposes portions of two different genes to encode a novel fusion protein with oncogenic function. The overexpressed genes or the novel fusion proteins may encode signal transduction proteins, growth factors, or, most frequently, transcription factors.

The translocations identified to date are seen most commonly with haematological malignancies. These translocations may be used to identify and classify different malignancies.

Translocation nomenclature *For example t(14:18)*. This relates to the chromosome number, that is chromosome 14 gains a fragment of chromosome 18; p refers to the short arm of chromosome, q to the long arm, further numbers relate to regions related to banding pattern of the chromosome. t(14:18)(q34;q:11) describes a translocation of chromosome 18 from the 11 region of the long arm on to the 34 region of the long arm of chromosome 14.

Examples of translocation *t(9:22)*. This is the Philadelphia chromosome which is seen in the leukaemias, principally chronic myeloid leukaemia (CML). It results in fusion of the *c-abl* gene on chromosome 9 to the *bcr* gene on chromosome 22, producing a novel protein with oncogenic properties. Numerous other translocations are seen in CML.

t(14:18). This is seen in 80% of follicular non-Hodgkin's lymphomas. It places the *bcl-2* gene under control of the immunoglobulin heavy chain (IgH) promoter. Overexpression of *bcl-2* leads to inhibition of apoptosis and clonal expansion of lymphocytes.

t(14:8). This is seen in Burkitt's lymphoma. It results in the *myc* gene on chromosome 8 being translocated to the IGH gene region on chromosome 14 giving abnormal overexpression of the *myc* oncogene.

t(11:22). This is seen in Ewing's sarcoma and results in production of a novel transcription factor.

Others. t(X:18) is associated with synovial sarcomas; t(2:13) has been seen in rhabdomyosarcomas.

Current issues

Screening PCR of the translocation point has been used to monitor response to therapy and predict relapse in certain malignancies. These molecular techniques are more sensitive than standard investigations of response.

CISPLATIN AND CARBOPLATIN

Cisplatin was identified as an anti-cancer drug in the early 1970s. Its activity against solid tumours encouraged its development as a widely prescribed chemotherapeutic agent despite significant toxicity. Carboplatin is a second generation analogue designed to avoid the non-haematological toxicity associated with cisplatin. Important differences in their activity mean that both drugs are still widely employed in the management of many solid tumours.

Uses

Cisplatin is a key agent in the combination treatment of germ cell tumours, especially testicular teratoma, resulting in complete response rates in excess of 90% with similar long-term survival. Clinical trials have suggested carboplatin is not as effective as cisplatin in the management of germ cell tumours.

Ovarian carcinoma is also highly sensitive to platinum-based chemotherapy. Platinum chemotherapy as a single agent or in combination with other drugs such as the alkylating agents is currently standard first line chemotherapy for ovarian epithelial malignancies. Whether full dose carboplatin is as effective as a cisplatin-containing combination is the focus of current clinical trials.

Cisplatin is also widely prescribed in the management of tumours of the bladder, breast, lung and head and neck. The experience in germ cell tumours has meant that the substitution of cisplatin for carboplatin is only justified following trials which confirm equal efficacy.

Mode of action

Cisplatin and carboplatin bind to DNA, RNA and protein, and form cross-links within the target molecule. The adducts formed with DNA are believed to be central to platinum drugs cytotoxicity.

Pharmacokinetics

Platinum drugs exist in both free and protein-bound forms within serum. Urinary excretion predominates with up to 35% of the total dose renally excreted within 24 hours. Careful assessment of renal function is therefore important prior to platinum administration.

Scheduling

Due to the potential renal toxicity of cisplatin, the drug should only be administered during an active diuresis. Pre-hydration to give a urine output of 100 ml per hour is followed by a 2–4 hour infusion of the drug. Post-hydration for up to 24 hours is required to maintain diuresis and thus reduce nephrotoxicity. Doses up to 100 mg/m² are given.

The dose of carboplatin is most frequently determined by direct correlation to the patients renal function using a standard formula, which relates to the predicted area under the curve (AUC) of carboplatin excretion but approximates to 400 mg/m². It does not require active diuresis and is therefore given as a short intravenous infusion.

Toxicity

1. Myelosupression. At standard doses cisplatin does not induce profound myelosuppression. A progressive anaemia of unknown cause is common and may require transfusion.

Carboplatin is dose limited by myelosuppression which occurs 14–21 days following IV administration. Severe, prolonged myelosuppression requires dose modification in subsequent cycles.

2. Nausea and vomiting. Cisplatin is invariably associated with profound nausea and vomiting. The development of the 5-HT3 antagonist anti-emetics, such as ondansetron, has dramatically improved the morbidity associated with this toxicity. Carboplatin is associated with much less severe nausea and vomiting, normally controlled with simple anti-emetics such as metoclopramide.

3. Alopecia. Cisplatin and carboplatin rarely induce alopecia.

4. Extravasation. Cisplatin and carboplatin are moderate vescicants and therefore require appropriate measures if extravasation occurs.

5. Nephrotoxicity. The dose-limiting toxicity of cisplatin is its nephrotoxicity. Cisplatin induces specific renal tubular damage to the distal convoluted tubule and collecting duct of the kidney. Adequate hydration greatly reduces this toxicity but cumulative damage may occur. The renal tubular damage can also induce renal magnesium wasting that may be both severe and permanent. Carboplatin induces minimal nephrotoxicity.

6. *Neurotoxicity.* A peripheral neuropathy principally affecting the sensory system occurs following repeated dosing. The neuropathy may recover partially over a period of months.

7. *Ototoxicity.* Cochlear damage rather than auditory nerve damage is believed to be responsible for the high-tone hearing loss associated with cisplatin. The effect is permanent. Pre-existing high-tone hearing damage precludes the use of cisplatin.

High dose

Haematological support with growth factors or stem-cell transfusions enables marked dose escalation of carboplatin. At these higher doses nephrotoxicity, neurotoxicity and hepatotoxicity predominate and are the dose-limiting side effects.

The renal and neurotoxicity of cisplatin prevents significant dose escalation.

Future directions

The development of other analogues of cisplatin with markedly reduced toxicities.

CLINICAL TRIALS

Oncology is a research-driven speciality with constant development of potential therapies. Although evidence-based medicine is important in all disciplines, rigorous testing of a new anti-cancer therapy is vital to establish both efficacy and toxicity before it becomes acceptable clinical practice. Clinical trials represent the final stage of a lengthy process (5–10 years) which involves initial *in vitro* studies and animal testing.

Trial design

Before embarking on a clinical trial, a clear statement of the trial's objectives, inclusion and exclusion criteria and data to be collected must be defined in a written protocol. This protocol should be strictly adhered to throughout the trial. A well-written protocol also includes background information (animal data, previous relevant trials), a management plan of all expected toxicities and dose modifications required. Statistical issues should be addressed.

Ethical committee approval of the protocol is mandatory in UK hospitals. Informed written consent is legally required to enter any patient into a clinical trial. Trials should comply with accepted codes of practice, for example GCP (Good Clinical Practice).

The assessment of any treatment, in particular a new drug, is performed in a number of well-defined 'phases'. These are as follows:

Phase I The aim of phase I studies is to determine toxicity (previously tested *in vitro* and in animals) and to establish the maximum tolerated dose (MTD). Disease response is not an endpoint. Dose escalation is performed, commencing at 10% of the LD10 in mice (the dose per m^2 that is lethal in 10% of mice). In general, three patients are treated at each dose level until side effects are seen, and then six patients per group until the maximum tolerated dose is reached. Dose escalation is calculated by one of several regimens; a modified Fabonicci formula is commonly used. Phase I trials of new anti-cancer treatments are performed on patients with any tumour, in whom no conventional therapy is appropriate. Patients must remain generally fit and, in particular, have near-normal renal and hepatic function. These trials are not randomized.

Phase II Once drug doses and scheduling have been defined from phase I trials, anti-tumour response can be studied in phase II trials. These can be randomized or nonrandomized studies (see below). The aim of phase II trials is therefore to assess the particular anti-tumour activity of a new treatment. In general, phase III studies are required to give conclusive results.

Phase III

Phase III studies are randomized trials comparing new with established treatments. The endpoints assessed may be response rates, survival, time to progression and/or quality of life. If the benefit of a new treatment is thought to be small, a large sample size will be required to achieve statistical significance. For this reason most of these trials are multi-centred.

Response endpoints

In order for results to be comparable across different centres, trial design must conform to accepted guidelines. These must include strict adherence to defined endpoints, including tumour response, survival, toxicity and quality of life.

Tumour response

The World Health Organization (WHO) defines tumour response rigidly:

1. Complete response. This implies the disappearance of all malignant disease for at least 4 weeks. It may be defined both clinically or pathologically, for example following 'second look' laparotomy.

2. Partial response. This is defined as a decrease in tumour size of at least 50% of the product of the tumour's longest dimension and its widest perpendicular measurement. This decrease in size must have a duration of at least 4 weeks without progressive disease elsewhere.

3. Stable disease. This is defined as a decrease in a tumour of less than 50%, or an increase in a tumour of less than 25% in the product of the measurable disease.

4. Progressive disease. This implies the presence of any new sites of disease or an increase of more than 25% in the product of the measurable disease.

5. Non-evaluable response. Frequently patients can not be classified according to the above criteria due to lack of data, loss of follow up, withdrawal or death. Exclusion of these patients from the trial introduces bias. The final analysis of trial data is therefore performed on an 'intention to treat' basis.

Survival

This is an important endpoint of many of the trials:

1. Overall survival. This is the length of time between entry to the trial and death from whatever cause.

2. Disease free survival. This is the time between entry into the trial and recurrence of the tumour or death from other causes.

3. Time to progression. This is the time between entry into the trial and disease progression or recurrence.

Toxicity

Toxicity is an important endpoint of trials and is usually classified according to the WHO toxicity criteria. Most drug side effects are classified according to four grades, with grade one being the least toxic and four the most toxic.

Quality of life

QL is increasingly being measured as a formal endpoint in many clinical trials. This is of particular importance in trials of palliative treatment.

Statistical analysis

Randomization

Randomization reduces bias by assigning individuals to each arm of the trial by chance alone. In most trials both the patient and the investigator are aware of the treatment they are having. Trials can however be 'blinded', where the patient or both the patient and the investigator are excluded from knowing the treatment that they are having.

Number of patients

The number of patients required in a trial is determined by the size of the effect under study and the statistical significance required. Therefore, to demonstrate a small effect at high significance, a large cohort of patients is required. However, to detect a 20% response rate of a new cancer treatment, as few as 14 patients are required: the probability of the first patient not responding to the drug is 0.8, the first two patients 0.64 (0.8×0.8) while the probability of all 14 patients failing is less than 0.05 $(= 0.8^{14})$. Therefore, if no responses are observed with 14 patients, the treatment can be assumed, with 95% confidence, to have a response rate less than 20%.

Survival curves

Survival data are generally presented graphically (Kaplan Meier curves) with the probability of survival plotted against time. The data presented can be actual survival, where follow-up data are complete for all patients, or actuarial, where patients are lost to follow-up. From these curves median survival and survival rates, for example 5 year survival, can be estimated.

Related topic of interest

Quality of life (p. 217)

COLORECTAL CANCER

Background

Incidence

Approximately 28 000 new cases are diagnosed each year in the UK. Colorectal carcinoma is the second most common malignancy after lung cancer, comprising 10–15% of all malignancies, and causes 19 000 deaths each year. Cancer of the colon is 1.5 times more common than rectal carcinoma

Risk factors

1. Diet. A diet rich in animal fats and meat and poor in fibre, common in Western countries, has been suggested as a cause for some colorectal cancers. This is reflected in the lower incidence in Africa, South America and Asia.

2. Inflammatory disease. There is an association with ulcerative colitis (cumulative risk of 7–15% at 20 years of disease) which is related to the extent of the bowel involvement and the duration of the inflammation. An association with Crohn's disease is controversial.

3. Familial association. Several familial conditions, which account for 5–10% of colorectal tumours, are described. These include hereditary non-polyposis coli (HNPCC), familial adenomatous polyposis coli and Gardner's syndrome. Specific gene defects associated with these conditions have been identified, for example mutations in the *APC* gene (5q21–22) (familial adenomatous polyposis coli) and mutations in DNA mismatch repair genes (HNPCC).

Aetiology

The progression from normal epithelium to hyperproliferative epithelium, benign adenoma, and ultimately invasive carcinoma of an individual lesion is well described. The stepwise accumulation of genetic defects associated with each of these lesions has also been demonstrated. *APC* mutations are associated with the development of benign adenomas whereas the progression to invasive carcinoma requires further mutations, for example *p53*, *DCC* and *RAS*.

These mutations may be caused by carcinogens present in faeces. Diets low in fibre prolong transit time and may prolong exposure to carcinogens. Bile salts are thought to act as carcinogens both directly and when degraded by bacteria present in the faeces.

Histology

Approximately 40% of large bowel cancers occur in the rectum, 20% in the sigmoid colon, 6% in the caecum and the rest in the remaining colon. Some 90–95% of tumours are adenocarcinomas, the histological types of cancer that occur are:

- Epithelial   adenocarcinoma (mucinous or signet ring)
  squamous cell carcinoma
  adenosquamous carcinoma undifferentiated.
- Carcinoid.
- Leiomyosarcoma.
- Primary malignant lymphoma.

These tumours are also described by their macroscopic appearance as either polypoid or sessile. Colorectal cancer normally disseminates by local invasion, lymphatic, venous and coelomic spread.

Clinical features

Presentation

Presentation can be with classical features of altered bowel habit, weight loss, rectal bleeding and vague abdominal pain, although the clinical features vary according to the site of the primary tumour and degree of spread. More occult tumours, typically of the right side of the colon and the caecum, can present with iron deficiency anaemia.

Investigations

A rectal examination is essential, three quarters of all rectal lesions can be felt by digital examination. Direct visualization of the bowel with rigid sigmoidoscopy (to 25 cm), flexible sigmoidoscopy and colonoscopy allows biopsy of suspicious lesions. Double contrast barium enema or CT may also provide a useful evaluation of the bowel.

Other investigations include measurement of the tumour marker CEA (carcino-embryonic antigen). Although elevation of this protein is not diagnostic it can be useful to monitor disease.

Staging

The Dukes' staging system (pathological staging) is used:

A   Confined to the bowel wall, that is mucosa and submucosa, or early muscular invasion.
B   Invasion through the muscle wall but no lymph node involvement.
C1 Lymph node involvement but not up to the highest point of vascular ligation.
C2 Nodes involved up to highest nodes at the point of ligation.
D   Distant metastases or advanced local disease.

The UICC staging system (TNM) can also be used:

Tis Carcinoma *in situ.*
T1   Tumour invades submucosa.
T2   Tumour invades through muscularis propia.
T3   Tumour invades through muscularis propia into subserosa or into non-peritonealized pericolic or perirectal tissues.
T4   Tumour perforates the visceral peritoneum or directly invades other organs or structures.

N1   Metastases in one to three pericolic or perirectal lymph nodes.
N2   Metastases in four or more pericolic or perirectal lymph nodes.
N3   Metastases in any lymph node along the course of a named vascular trunk.

M1   Distant metastases.

Management

Surgery

Radical resection is the standard operation for primary colorectal carcinoma because of the risk of unsuspected nodal metastases. Patients with early stage colorectal carcinoma are usually cured by surgical resection alone. The long-term results with rectal carcinoma are related to the initial surgical resection.

Surgery may also be indicated in patients with advanced disease. Resection of isolated liver metastases in addition to the primary may be beneficial. Further resection of a local recurrence is associated with improved long-term survival.

Surgery may be used in the palliative setting to manage or prevent an obstructing lesion.

Radiotherapy

Radiotherapy is used in the treatment of rectal carcinomas. It is not commonly used in the management of colon cancers because of the toxicity to adjacent organs. Adjuvant radiotherapy is indicated in high-risk rectal carcinomas before or following total resection. Local recurrences can be palliated with radiotherapy. Metastatic bone disease may respond to palliative radiotherapy.

Chemotherapy

Adjuvant chemotherapy for high-risk colorectal carcinoma has become accepted practice. It is now used routinely for Dukes' C carcinoma; 6 months adjuvant treatment with 5-FU may increase long-term survival from 40 to 60%. Current trials assess the role of adjuvant chemotherapy for Dukes' B carcinoma. 5-FU is the most active agent in colorectal carcinoma with a response rate of approximately 25%. In combination with folinic acid or levamisole responses rates of up to 40% have been demonstrated.

Second-line treatment of relapsed cases is disappointing. Mitomycin C is used but with response rates of approximately 15%.

Prognostic factors

Stage of tumour

Stage A 80% 5 year survival.
Stage B 50% 5 year survival.
Stage C1 40% 5 year survival.
Stage C2 12% 5 year survival.
Stage D 5% 5 year survival.

Age	Age below 40 is an adverse prognostic factor, possibly reflecting a biologically more aggressive tumour.

Screening

Screening of high-risk individuals, for example those with extensive inflammatory bowel disease or known familial predisposition, is performed. Following resection of a primary lesion, annual colonoscopy is recommended.

The role of screening of the general population is controversial. Faecal occult blood testing of average-risk populations has recently demonstrated a reduction of mortality between 15–18%. This is not routine practice currently.

Current issues

Adjuvant therapy	The role of adjuvant chemotherapy for Dukes' B carcinoma is being addressed in the QUASAR (Quick and Simple and Reliable) trial. Trials of monoclonal antibodies also in the adjuvant setting are being conducted.
Molecular mechanisms	The molecular pathways of carcinogenesis are being elucidated. Their prognostic significance and possible therapeutic implications are also being investigated.

Further reading

Williams S. *et al.* In: Peckham M, Pinedo H, Veroneri U, eds. *Oxford Textbook of Oncology*. Oxford University Press, 1995; 1133–68.

Related topics of interest

Familial cancer syndromes (p. 92)
Tumour markers (p. 263)

CYCLOPHOSPHAMIDE

Cyclophosphamide is the most frequently used alkylating agent. Other alkylating agents include ifosfamide, nitrogen mustard, chlorambucil, melphalan, thiotepa and busulphan. These drugs share a common mechanism of action but have different toxicities and clinical efficacies.

Uses

Cyclophosphamide is frequently used in combination with other chemotherapeutic drugs in the treatment of lymphomas, small cell lung cancer, breast carcinoma and ovarian carcinoma.

Cyclophosphamide and other alkylating agents are frequently employed in high-dose chemotherapy regimes as their principal toxicity is haematological. Cyclophosphamide is also be used to mobilize haematopoietic stem cells into the peripheral circulation for collection and later administration following high-dose myelo-ablative chemotherapy.

Cyclophosphamide is also used as an immunosuppressant in the treatment of non-malignant disease such as rheumatoid arthritis and other connective tissue disorders.

Mode of action

Cyclophosphamide is a pro-drug activated by hepatic metabolism to cytotoxic metabolites (e.g. phosphoramide mustard). These bind to DNA, causing cross-linkage or breaks in double-stranded DNA which lead to cell death. Cyclophosphamide, like other alkylating agents, is most active against rapidly dividing cells.

Pharmacokinetics

Following hepatic metabolism of cyclophosphamide, many of the metabolites are renally excreted. The metabolism and excretion show marked inter-patient variability. Certain metabolites (acrolein) may lead to a haemorrhagic cystitis. This may be prevented with the concurrent administration of MESNA which, in the urine, binds and inactivates toxic metabolites. Renal impairment leads to an accumulation of the toxic metabolites and therefore prolongs the drugs cytotoxicity. Hepatic failure is also associated with prolongation of the drug's half-life.

Scheduling

Cyclophosphamide is given both orally and systemically. The dose given is dependent on the tumour type, stage and general condition of the patient. Typical combination regimes include a single bolus dose of cyclophosphamide 3 weekly in a dose of approximately 750 mg/m^2. Prolonged oral administration (14 days) reduces the toxicity associated with peak plasma concentrations.

Dose escalation is possible with appropriate haematological support such as growth factors or stem cell transfusions. With high-dose chemotherapy pulmonary, cardiac and renal toxicities are more frequent.

Toxicity

1. Myelosuppression. Cyclophosphamide produces dose-limiting myelosuppression (especially leukopenia). The nadir following bolus systemic administration typically occurs after approximately 10 days, with count recovery by 14–21 days.

2. Nausea and vomiting. Alkylating agents induce nausea and vomiting in a dose-dependent manner. 5-HT3 antagonist anti-emetics are frequently employed in addition to metoclopramide and steroids.

3. Alopecia. This occurs in a proportion of patients. It is an inevitable consequence of high-dose treatment

4. Extravasation. Alkylating agents are moderate vesicants and therefore require appropriate measures if extravasation occurs.

5. Gonadal failure. The effect on sterility is dose dependent. Standard doses usually lead to a reversible decrease in fertility. High doses may induce permanent sterility. Counselling is therefore of paramount importance and sperm storage should be offered routinely.

6. Neurological. Although cyclophosphamide is rarely neurotoxic, ifosfamide may induce confusion, depression, hysteria and altered levels of consciousness in up to 30% of patients. It is particularly associated with hepatic dysfunction.

7. Pulmonary. Pulmonary fibrosis and pneumonitis can occur with prolonged administration.

8. Haemorrhagic cystitis. Cyclophosphamide induces this in up to 10% of patients. The concurrent administration of adequate hydration and MESNA reduces this toxicity.

9. Cardiac toxicity. High-dose cyclophosphamide may be associated with acute cardiac necrosis.

10. Secondary malignancies. Alkylating agents induce DNA damage and therefore secondary malignancies, such as leukaemias, may result.

DOXORUBICIN AND EPIRUBICIN

Doxorubicin is a naturally derived antibiotic with cytotoxic and hence anti-tumour activity. Other synthetic anthracyclines such as epirubicin and idarubicin have been developed in an attempt to reduce the toxicity profile.

Uses	Doxorubicin is frequently used in combination regimes to treat a variety of malignancies, including breast carcinoma, lymphomas, sarcomas, lung carcinomas and haematological malignancies. It is the single most active agent in the treatment of breast cancer.
Mode of action	The exact mechanism of action of doxorubicin has not been fully elucidated, but it can bind tightly to DNA and once intercalated inhibits DNA replication. Topoisomerase II (the enzyme responsible for unwinding the double helix of DNA prior to replication) is inhibited, causing DNA-strand breaks and thus preventing replication. It is mainly effective against cells in the S phase of the cell cycle.
Pharmacokinetics	Doxorubicin is rapidly cleared from the plasma, metabolized in the liver and excreted into the bile duct. This needs to be taken into account in hepatic impairment as toxicity will be exacerbated. Renal excretion is minimal ($<10\%$). 75% of the drug is protein-bound and penetration of the CSF is poor.
Scheduling	*Intravenous.* Injected as a bolus into fast running drips, this is the most frequently used route of administration. Single bolus doses every 3 weeks are commonly used; divided doses may have greater efficacy, but are associated with greater toxicity.
	Intravesical. Direct instillation of doxorubicin into the bladder is used in management of superficial bladder carcinoma.
	Intra-arterial. Intra-arterial perfusion of doxorubicin permits local perfusion with high levels of the drug without associated systemic toxicity.
Toxicity	*1. Myelosupression.* This is the dose-limiting toxicity with a nadir at 10–14 days after treatment; leucocytes are primarily affected.

2. *Nausea and vomiting*. This can be severe but is controlled in the majority of patients with anti-emetic combinations.

3. *Gastrointestinal*. Mucositis is a common side effect. An oral burning sensation may precede ulceration; repeat administration without dose modification should be avoided.

4. *Alopecia*. This occurs in all patients, but is transient and hair returns following the completion of treatment. Scalp cooling during administration may have a role in lessening hair loss.

5. *Extravasation*. The anthracyclines are highly vesicant and cause tissue necrosis when extravasated.

6. *Cardiac toxicity*. Doxorubicin may be associated with cardiac toxicity manifested as arrhythmias, heart failure and ECG changes. Severe cardiac failure may occur suddenly. Toxicity is dose-dependent: a cumulative dose greater than 550 mg/m^2 should be avoided. Epirubicin causes less cardiac toxicity than doxorubicin.

7. *Radiosensitizer*. Anthracyclines sensitize cells to the effects radiation. Their use prior to radiotherapy is therefore contra-indicated.

8. *Others*. Doxorubicin is red in solution and may lead to discolouration of the urine.

High dose

The cardiac toxicity of the anthracyclines prevents dose escalation in high-dose combinations.

DRUG RESISTANCE

Despite the continual discovery of novel chemotherapeutic agents, the majority of tumours remain incurable once they become metastatic. Many tumours that initially respond to treatment later relapse. Drug resistance of a fraction of the initial tumour burden creates a major obstacle in the treatment of the majority of haematological and solid malignancies.

Most chemotherapy regimes employed today have evolved in an attempt to overcome drug resistance. Using cytotoxic drugs with differing mechanisms of action may prevent the selection of resistant cell populations.

Tumour cell resistance to chemotherapy may be classified as either primary or secondary.

Primary resistance

Tumours that demonstrate primary resistance fail to respond to chemotherapy from the start. This may be due to the following:

Apparent resistance	This may be due to inadequate dosing, inappropriate route of administration or poor compliance.
Physiological resistance	The relative hypoxia of tumour cells may lead to anaerobic glycolysis and an acidic environment within the tumour bed. This directly decreases the efficacy of chemotherapy and radiotherapy.
Biological resistance	Tumours are generally made up of a number of sub-populations of cells with different genetic and hence phenotypic characteristics. Sensitivity to drug treatment may therefore vary in different regions of the tumour.
Pharmacological resistance	This may be due to, for example, poor penetration of drugs through the blood–brain barrier or into the testes.

Secondary resistance

Secondary or acquired drug resistance follows exposure of cells to chemotherapy. The mechanisms by which tumour cells become resistant to chemotherapy on the whole reflect the physiological processes required by normal cells/tissues to handle toxic metabolites/substances. Tumour cells that demonstrate secondary resistance are selected by their survival advantage. One or a combination of these mechanisms may be active in a tumour cell.

Mechanisms of acquired drug resistance include:

Increased drug extrusion

P-glycoprotein (Pgp) is a plasma-membrane protein coded for by the *mdr* gene. Pgp functions as an energy-dependent molecular efflux pump in normal cells which actively extrudes drugs from tumour cells, thereby preventing them from reaching their molecular site of action. Overexpression of Pgp leads to resistance to a wide range of naturally occurring cytotoxic agents, for example doxorubicin, daunorubicin, vincristine, vinblastine, Taxol, etoposide and mitomycin, a phenotype known as multi-drug resistance (MDR).

Several agents have been identified that reverse MDR related drug resistance through competitive inhibition of the membrane pump, for example verapamil, cyclosporin A, tamoxifen, quinidine, progesterone and trifluoperazine. These drugs have an additive inhibitory effect. Combinations of more than one drug may therefore prevent toxicity.

Decreased drug uptake

Certain drugs enter the cell via an active-transport mechanism. Loss or inactivation of this transport system is one of the causes of methotrexate resistance.

Decreased drug activation

Several drugs require metabolic activation to exert their effects. Alterations in the levels of the activating enzymes reduce levels of active agent and lessen efficacy. 6-Mercaptopurine (6-MP) requires enzymatic conversion to an active form; resistance to 6-MP is associated with decreased enzymatic conversion.

Increased drug inactivation

Several anti-cancer drugs cause cellular damage via free radical production. A number of protective mechanisms exist within cells to render these toxins less harmful, for example glutathiones and metallothionines. An increase in the activity of these systems may lead to reduced efficacy.

Alteration in DNA repair mechanisms

Many agents ultimately express their action through DNA damage and a presumed induction of apoptosis. An increased ability to repair DNA protects against this and thus induces resistance. Several mechanisms exist.

Alkylguanine-DNA alklyltransferase. This is an important component of cellular DNA repair pathways. It protects the cell from the mutagenic and carcinogenic effects of alkylating agents by removing adducts which enable cross linking between DNA strands.

Topoisomerase 1 and 2. These produce controlled single- and double-strand breaks in DNA translation, synthesis and repair. These breaks help to unravel and separate knotted strands of DNA. Inhibitors prevent this vital action and ultimately lead to cell death. Chemoresistance occurs in cells that develop structural changes in these enzymes to circumvent inhibitor activity.

Increased drug tolerance
A number of different mechanisms exist. An example of this is the induction of asparagine synthetase allowing the cell to produce its own asparagine. Normal cells are unable to synthesise asparagine. Asparaginase hydrolyses asparagine, and without this the cell cannot survive.

Conclusion

Many solid tumours initially respond to chemotherapy treatment. However, the selection of resistant cells ultimately leads to progression, with disease refractory to treatment. Chemotherapy practice has developed over the last 10 years in an attempt to prevent this and a variety of methods are increasingly used in clinical practice. Higher doses, more intensive chemotherapy, MDR modulators and enzyme inhibitors may become commonplace in the clinical setting of cancer chemotherapy. Although benefits have been shown in some tumour groups, in many malignancies these have failed to improve long-term survival.

ENDOCRINE TUMOURS

Malignant endocrine tumours may affect the exocrine glands of the pancreas, the adrenal, parathyroid, thyroid or pituitary gland. Malignancies may also arise in the neuroendocrine cells of tissues not usually associated with an endocrine function.

Carcinoid tumours

Carcinoid tumours are generally slow-growing malignant tumours occurring predominantly in people under 50.

Histology

Carcinoid tumours arise from neuroendocrine cells, most frequently within the small bowel, appendix and descending colon. Metastases occur frequently (except from an appendiceal origin), mainly to the liver, but also to lung and bone. Carcinoid tumours can secrete 5-hydroxytryptamine (5-HT; serotonin), bradykinins, prostaglandins and/or histamine.

Clinical features

Carcinoid may present with symptoms related to the effect of local tumour growth or metastatic disease. In less than 10% of carcinoid tumours, the secretion of active inflammatory mediators into the systemic circulation may produce a complex of typical symptoms known as carcinoid syndrome. The failure of normal hepatic metabolism of these factors implies either hepatic metastases from a GI primary or a bronchial or other extra-GI primary. 5-HT secretion produces diarrhoea, hypertension and, in the long term, endocardial fibrosis which may lead to tricuspid regurgitation. Bradykinin and prostaglandin secretion leads to facial flushing and oedema. Histamine release produces in bronchospasm, skin wheals and lacrimation.

Investigation

5-HIAA. Twenty-four hour urinary 5-hydroxyindolacetic acid (HIAA), a normal degradation of 5-HT, is elevated.

MIBG scan. Assessment of radiolabelled meta-iodo-benzyl-guanidine (MIBG) uptake is useful in cases where there is no appreciable excess of urinary 5-HIAA, and for assessing the extent of metastatic disease if resection is contemplated.

Hepatic arteriography. This is performed pre-operatively if palliative excision of liver metastases is planned.

Management

Treatment of carcinoid tumours usually involves radical surgery of both primary and occasionally of metastatic disease. Octreotide may improve diarrhoea and flushing. Response rates of approximately 30% are possible with streptozotocin-based chemotherapy regimes. However, these are of short duration and produce no overall increase in survival. Embolization or ligation of the hepatic artery may also be used to treat hepatic metastases.

Prognosis

Localized carcinoid tumour amenable to surgery is associated with an excellent prognosis (approximately 95% 5 year survival). The presence of distant metastatic disease is associated with a 5 year survival less than 20%.

Islet tumours of the pancreas

Islet tumours of the pancreas are uncommon and comprise a diverse group of hormone-secreting tumours.

Insulinoma

These are derived from the β cells of the pancreas; 10% are malignant. They present with hypoglycaemia in approximately 80% of patients. Investigation demonstrates fasting hypoglycaemia in the presence an inappropriately high level of insulin and elevated pro-insulin levels in 90% of patients. Partial pancreatectomy may be performed for localized disease. For unresectable or metastatic disease systemic chemotherapy with streptozotocin with 5-FU and/or doxorubicin has a 50–60% response rate. Biological therapy with interferon-α may also be beneficial.

Glucagonoma

These arise from the α cells of the islets. Sixty per cent are malignant, and they are generally slow-growing. They are frequently associated with a characteristic migratory necrolytic skin rash at presentation. Management usually involves surgery, with chemotherapy reserved for treatment of metastatic cases. The skin rash may improve with the use of octreotide to suppress glucagon secretion.

Gastrinoma	Gastrinomas arise most frequently in the pancreas or duodenum. They are usually malignant, with 60% showing metastases at diagnosis, usually to the liver or lymph nodes. Excessive gastrin secretion leads to recurrent severe peptic ulceration (Zollinger–Ellison syndrome). Diarrhoea is seen in 30–50% of cases. Investigations reveal elevated gastrin. With frequent metastatic disease, surgery is rarely useful as a mode of treatment. H_2-receptor antagonists may control acid secretion. Prognosis is relatively good, despite the high rate of metastases, with 80% 5 year survival.
Others	These include VIPoma and somatostatinoma.

Adrenal tumours

Adrenal cortex

Incidence. Malignant tumours of the adrenal cortex are rare, with less than 100 deaths per year in the UK.

Histology. Most malignant tumours are carcinomas, but anaplastic tumours do occur.

Clinical features. Approximately 50% of malignant tumours are functional, secreting corticosteroids or sex hormone. They may therefore manifest features of excess hormone secretion, for example Cushing's syndrome, virilization or feminization. Approximately 70% of patients have metastases at presentation, usually to lymph nodes, lung or liver.

Investigation. This involves the measurement of serum and urinary hormone levels, ultrasound and CT imaging. MRI can help to distinguish between adenomas and malignant tumours.

Management. The treatment of choice is radical surgical excision, which can be curative in limited disease. Debulking surgery has a role in controlling hormone secretion and local morbidity. In metastatic or recurrent disease, Mitotane has a 33% response rate and reduces secreted hormone levels. Palliation of hormone effects can be achieved with metyrapone and aminoglutethamide. Chemotherapy with cisplatin or etoposide may be effective.

Prognosis. This depends on the degree of differentiation and stage at presentation; median survival for anaplastic cancer is 5 months; it is 40 months for differentiated carcinomas.

Adrenal medulla

Tumours of the adrenal medulla are most frequently phaeochromocytomas; 10% of these are malignant and 10% are bilateral (10% are extra-adrenal).

Incidence. The peak incidence is in the 35–55 age range.

Histology. The tumours arise from neuro-endocrine chromaffin cells within the adrenal medulla.

Clinical features. Both benign and malignant phaeochromocytoma usually present with symptoms of hypertension (either paroxysmal or persistent), with headaches, postural hypotension, palpitations, pallor, sweating, tremor and chest pain, and feelings of apprehension.

Investigations. Twenty-four hour urinary vanillyl-mandelic acid (VMA) is raised in 85% of patients. Urinary catecholamines such as adrenaline, noradrenaline and dopamine may also be elevated. In addition to CT or MRI scanning, a radiolabelled meta-iodobenzylguanidine (MIBG) scan may be performed to identify extra-adrenal or metastatic disease.

Management. Surgery may be used to resect primary and recurrent disease. In patients not fit for surgery, symptom control may be achieved with phenoxybenzamine (an α-adrenergic receptor antagonist). Chemotherapy is infrequently used in the management of malignant phaeochromocytoma; cyclophosphamide, vincristine and dacarbazine may produce some response. Higher doses of radiolabelled MIBG may be used as palliative therapy in tumours which actively uptake a test dose.

Prognosis. For malignant phaeochromocytoma prognosis is poor, with very few long-term survivors.

Parathyroid tumours

Malignant parathyroid tumours are very rare representing only 5% all parathyroid tumours. However, they are important contributors to the various types of multiple endocrine neoplasia (MEN) syndromes (see below).

The tumours are usually functional, secreting parathyroid hormone, and resulting in the features of hyperparathyroidism, with hypercalcaemia, hypophosphataemia and a hyperchloraemic metabolic acidosis. Spread is most often to the lungs and liver.

Multiple endocrine neoplasia

Of the endocrine tumours mentioned above, it is a common phenomenon to find the co-existence of several endocrine tumours within the same individual. These can often involve a mixture of malignant tumours and hyperplastic tissues or benign adenomata. Several patterns are recognized:

MEN type I (Werner's syndrome)	Werner's syndrome usually includes a parathyroid and pancreatic tumour (in 95 and 80% of cases, respectively) and/or pituitary (65%), adrenal cortical (40%) or carcinoid tumours. A candidate gene, *MEN1*, located on chromsome 11 (q13), has recently been identified. Loss of heterozygosity at 11q13 is a frequent finding in many endocrine malignancies.
MEN type II (Sipple's disease)	Sipple's disease also has a genetic basis, being inherited in an autosomal dominant Mendelian fashion. It can be divided into two, sub-groups. MENIIA includes parathyroid tumours, phaeochromocytoma and medullary cancer of the thyroid. Type IIB may have additional subcutaneous or submucosal neuronal tumours, autonomic ganglio-neuromatosis and Marfanoid features.
MEN type III (mixed)	This type also involves phaeochromocytoma and medullary cancer of the thyroid, but parathyroid tumours are absent and neuromata around the lips, tongue and GI tract are present. Patients often exhibit hyper-extensible joints, pes cavus and prognathia.

Related topics of interest

Brain tumours (p. 21)
Thyroid cancer (p. 259)

EXTRAVASATION

Extravasation is a serious complication of intravenous administration of cytotoxic drugs. It can be defined as the inadvertent or inappropriate administration of drugs or fluids subcutaneously or subdermally, rather than via the intended, intravenous route. It should be an avoidable side-effect in the majority of cases.

Incidence   Administration of intravenous substances, including crystalloid fluids and antibiotics is associated with extravasation in 20–30% of cases. If the same cannula is used for 7 days, the incidence is as high as 95%. The rate is much lower for cytotoxic agents, partly because infusion times are usually relatively short, and also partly because of awareness of the greater potential for harm.

Effects   Extravasation of cytotoxic drugs can lead to severe damage. This can lead to cosmetically damaging tissue necrosis and damage to underlying structures such as tendons. The result can be significant loss of function for the patient and may require reconstructive surgery.

Prevention   A few basic principles can minimize the occurrence of extravasation:

1. Awareness of the problem. This is important not just on the part of those administering the drugs, but also on the part of those receiving them. Patients must be warned of symptoms for which they should be vigilant.

2. Careful choice of cannula site and type. For certain high-risk drugs, or for long infusions, an in-dwelling central line (Hickman line) may be best.

3. Skilled insertion of cannula. Staff administering the drugs should be adequately trained, specifically in the administration of cytotoxics. GTN patches can be useful to dilate veins in a patient who is difficult to cannulate.

4. Regular assessment of the cannula. Prior to cytotoxic administration the cannula should be assessed to ensure it remains patent.

5. Careful administration. Cytotoxics should be administered with great caution.

6. Warning. IN DOUBT, STOP THE INFUSION.

| Diagnosis | If extravasation does occur, early diagnosis and prompt management are essential for a good outcome. Educate patients to recognize and encourage administering staff to enquire about symptoms such as: |

- Burning, stinging pain.
- Altered appearance of the skin: erythema, swelling, or induration.
- Leakage of fluid from around the cannula site.

Extravasation should also be suspected if it is not possible to:
- Obtain free flow through the cannula from a fast-running bag of saline.
- Inject a bolus of saline solution without resistance.
- Aspirate blood via the cannula.

Management

When extravasation is suspected, prompt action is essential, ideally within the hour, and certainly in less than 24 hours. A 'watch and wait' policy is not appropriate, as it may take many weeks for the full extent of damage to be appreciated. An extravasation kit, which includes a list of the classification of cytotoxic drugs according to their necrotic potential, and contains all the appropriate substances for these treatments should be available in any location where chemotherapy is administered.

Once the extravasated drug has been identified, specific management should be given dictated by the potential of the drug to cause tissue damage.

| Vesicants | These drugs are associated with severe local necrosis and may require plastic surgery. |

1. Vinca alkaloids. These include vincristine, vinblastine and vindesine.
- Immediately stop the infusion, aspirate the remaining drug and 3–4 ml blood, mark the area and remove the cannula.
- Spread and dilute vesicant: inject hyaluronidase, an enzyme that leads to the reversible breakdown of the extracellular matrix enhancing permeation of the drug and promoting resorption of tissue fluid. Aspirate any fluid that collects.
- Apply a warm compress for 24 hours with a 30 minute break every 3 hours.
- Elevate, encourage exercise and inspect the affected area for erythema, induration, blitering or necrosis. Provide adequate analgesia.

	• A review should be carried out by a plastic surgery specialist for consideration of open drainage.
Anthracyclines and others	Danorubucin, doxorubucin, epirubucin, mitomycin C, actinomycin D, streptozocin, Carmustine (BCNU), Dacarbazine, Paciltaxel (Taxol), Docetaxel (Taxotere), cisplatin.

<table without borders below>

Anthracyclines and others Danorubucin, doxorubucin, epirubucin, mitomycin C, actinomycin D, streptozocin, Carmustine (BCNU), Dacarbazine, Paciltaxel (Taxol), Docetaxel (Taxotere), cisplatin.

- Immediately stop infusion, aspirate remaining drug and 3–4 ml blood, mark area and remove cannula.
- Localize and neutralize vesicant: inject hydrocortisone 100 mg IV via new cannula and 100 mg in 6–8 aliquots around region of extravasation.
- Apply cold compress for 24 hours with a 30 minute break every 3 hours.
- Elevate, encourage exercise and inspect affected area for erythema, induration, blistering or necrosis; provide adequate analgesia.
- Apply 1% hydrocortisone cream if inflammation present.
- For anthracyclines only: apply DMSO qds for 7 days.
- Review by a plastic surgery specialist for consideration of open drainage.

Irritants/non-vesicants Extravasation of irritants (carboplatin, etoposide, methotroxate and mitoxantrone) or drugs classified as non-vesicants (5-FU, cyclophosphamide, ifosfamide, bleomycin, melphalan, thiotepa, cytarabine, asparaginase, gemcitabine) should receive careful assessment and management.

- Immediately stop infusion, aspirate remaining drug and 3–4 ml blood, mark area and remove cannula.
- Elevate, encourage exercise and inspect affected area for erythema, induration, blistering or necrosis.
- Provide adequate analgesia.

Related topic of interest

Chemotherapy – (d) complications (p. 58)

FAMILIAL CANCER SYNDROMES

Incidence

Inherited cancer accounts for 5–10% of malignancies. Clinical features that suggest the presence of an inherited familial syndrome include early age of onset, a variety of different primary tumours within the family or a family history that fits into a recognized syndrome.

Aetiology

The genetic abnormalities of cancer lead to abnormal overexpression or loss of function of specific gene products. Most cancers require multiple genetic abnormalities which finally lead to the malignant phenotype. In most cancers these are probably acquired by somatic mutation. In familial cancers, inheritance of germline mutations in one or more of the same carcinogenic genes leads to a predisposition to cancer.

Investigation of familial cancer syndromes has lead to the identification of the specific inherited mutated genes that play a role in carcinogenesis. Many of these genetic abnormalities have subsequently been identified in sporadic cancers where the defects occur by somatic mutation.

Several of these inherited syndromes can predispose to more than one tumour type. The first of these genes to be identified was the *Rb* gene in familial retinoblastoma. The inherited defective gene has also been identified in familial adenomatous polyposis coli, some familial breast cancer, the Li–Fraumeni syndrome and familial melanoma among others.

Inherited cancer syndromes

Li–Fraumeni syndrome

This is caused by a germline mutation of the *p53* gene. The family members have a high chance of early onset (early adult life) cancers including osteosarcomas, soft-tissue sarcomas, gliomas and breast cancer.

Familial adenomatous polyposis coli

This is an autosomal dominant condition characterized by multiple adenomatous polyps of the colon that appear at an early age. This condition is caused by mutations in the *APC* gene (5q21–22). The exact function of this tumour-suppressor gene is unclear, but it plays a role in cell–cell contact.

Hereditary non-polyposis colorectal carcinoma	HNPCC includes site-specific colorectal cancer (Lynch syndrome I) and the cancer family syndrome (Lynch syndrome II). Lynch syndrome I is characterized by an autosomal dominant susceptibility to colorectal carcinoma, with an early age of onset and a high frequency of primary colonic carcinomas. Lynch syndrome II has all the features of Lynch syndrome I but it is also associated with extracolonic carcinomas particularly carcinoma of the endometrium and ovary. HNPCC is caused by mutations in DNA mismatch repair genes. HNPCC syndromes may account for 5–10% of all colorectal carcinomas.
Familial breast/ovarian cancer	Familial predisposition to early onset breast cancer and ovarian cancer is associated with germline mutations in the *BRCA1* gene. Less than 5% of patients with breast cancer will have germline mutations in this gene that can be passed on to offspring. The function of this gene has yet to be fully characterized. *BRCA2* is an unrelated gene which is mutated in other cases of familial breast cancer.
Others	Several other familial syndromes have been identified, and new gene defects are constantly being delineated.

Genetic counselling

Genetic counselling in these families includes a careful determination of the family tree. This enables advice regarding future risk in patients' families to be given. At present, genetic testing of specific mutations is rarely performed. As the gene defects in these conditions are characterized, a more accurate assessment of risk may be possible following DNA analysis.

The identification of increased risk from such genetic counselling enables more vigilant screening to be instigated, for example regular colonoscopy, early mammography. The role of therapeutic preventative measures such as bilateral mastectomies in BRCA1 families is controversial. A trial of aspirin to prevent colon cancer in HNPCC families is currently underway.

Current issues

Genetic testing of individuals for specific cancer gene mutations is now possible. However, in the absence of an appropriate intervention, the psychological and social effect of such testing is unclear. The implications for future insurance and employment prospects are controversial.

5-FLUOROURACIL

5-Fluorouracil (5-FU) is a fluorinated pyrimidine anti-metabolite. It was designed in the 1950s and as such represents one of the first rationally designed anti-tumour agents.

Uses

5-FU as a single agent is prescribed extensively in the management of colorectal carcinoma both as an adjuvant treatment and in the palliative setting. As a single agent a response rate of approximately 20% can be achieved. This can be increased to 30–40% by the use of agents which modulate 5-FU's metabolism and thus enhance its cytotoxic action.

In combination with other drugs, 5-FU is also prescribed in the management of a wide variety of primary tumours, including breast, gastric and head and neck cancer.

Mode of action

5-FU is an analogue of uracil, a pyrimidine base essential to nucleic acid metabolism. The fluorinated nature of 5-FU interferes with the activity and metabolism of the nucleotide metabolites. 5-FU requires enzymatic conversion to one of these nucleotides to become active and is therefore a pro-drug. The metabolites interfere with both DNA and RNA synthesis and may also directly interfere with protein synthesis. Inhibition of the key enzyme thymidylate synthetase (TS) also inhibits DNA synthesis.

Pharmacokinetics

5-FU is not routinely given orally because its absorption following oral administration is erratic and incomplete. 5-FU metabolism occurs in all tissues, although predominantly in the liver (80%) with only 15% of the drug being excreted unchanged in the urine.

Following IV administration, the half-life of 5-FU is only 10 minutes and it is undetectable in the serum after 2 hours. 5-FU may be given as a continuous infusion to maintain serum levels and theoretically enhance the cytotoxicity.

Hepatic metabolism enables higher doses to be given by direct intra-hepatic infusion. This may deliver a greater cytotoxicity effect to liver metastases with no increase in systemic levels and hence toxicity.

Leucovorin (folinic acid). The metabolism of 5-FU and its metabolites may be altered to enhance the cytotoxicity of the drug. Leucovorin stabilizes the metabolites which cause TS inhibition, prolonging 5-FU's half-life

Scheduling

5-FU may be given as an IV injection, an intra-arterial injection and as a continuous ambulatory IV infusion prolonged over many months using portable pumps.

Toxicity

5-FU is well tolerated, with minimal toxicity, and thus is used extensively in the palliative setting.

1. Myelosuppression. Along with GI toxicity this is the predominant toxicity following bolus administration. It is less common with continuous infusions. The nadir tends to occur 7–14 days following administration. A megaloblastic anaemia may follow prolonged administration.

2. GI toxicity. Mucositis affecting the whole GI tract can occur. Angular stomatitis and oral ulceration should lead to discontinuation of infusional treatment and a reduction of dose once symptoms have settled. The use of allopurinol mouth wash may alleviate these symptoms. Persistent diarrhoea may occur and should also lead to a reduction in dose.

3. Nausea and vomiting. Although potentially a problem, many patients require no anti-emetics.

4. Alopecia. Total alopecia rarely occurs but many patients experience some degree of hair loss.

5. Ischaemic heart disease. Angina and, rarely, myocardial infarction may be caused by 5-FU. Although the precise mechanism is unknown, it is believed to be related to coronary artery spasm. Chest pain, in patients receiving 5-FU, should be assessed to be determine whether it is ischaemic in nature.

6. Cerebellar toxicity. A cerebellar syndrome with ataxia, slurred speech and nystagmus occurs rarely. It is associated with high peak levels and therefore more likely with bolus injection based regimes. It is generally reversible and symptoms improve when the 5-FU is discontinued.

7. *Palmar plantar erythema.* Erythema of the palms of the hands and soles of the feet is seen at higher doses which can be painful. It is treated with pyridoxine (50 mg tds). If this is unsuccessful the changes are reversible on stopping or reducing the dose of 5-FU.

GASTRIC CANCER

Background

Incidence

There are 12 000 new cases of gastric carcinoma diagnosed in the UK each year with a male to female ratio of 3:2. It is the fifth commonest cause of cancer death in the UK accounting for 10% of all cancer-related deaths. The incidence of gastric carcinoma world-wide has been falling over the last 50 years.

Risk factors

1. Diet. The risk is increased with certain foods such as smoked, salted or poorly preserved food. Diets rich in fruit and vegetables reduce the risk.

2. Smoking. Associated with up to three-fold increased risk.

3. Genetic. Positive family history increases the risk two- to three-fold. Blood group A is associated with an increased risk.

4. Geographical. The Japanese have an increased risk, falling with migration to low-risk areas.

5. Chronic atrophic gastritis. This leads to intestinal metaplasia, dysplasia and ultimately malignancy. It is seen in the elderly, those with pernicious anaemia and in the gastric remnant following gastrectomy.

6. Helicobacter. Helicobacter pylori infection is associated with an increased risk.

7. Social class. Increased risk in lower social classes.

Aetiology

N-nitroso compounds, formed by the action of gastric bacteria on nitrates occurring in food, are thought to be carcinogenic.

A number of genetic abnormalities have been linked to gastric carcinoma including allelic deletions of the *MCC* (mutated in colorectal cancer), *APC* (adenomatous polyposis coli) and *p53* tumour-suppressor genes.

Histology

More than 90% of stomach cancers are adenocarcinomas, sub-divided into an intestinal type and a diffuse type:

1. The intestinal type. This is characterized by cohesive neoplastic cells forming glandular structures. It usually occurs in the distal stomach, in elderly patients, and can be ulcerative or polypoid. It is often associated with intestinal metaplasia.

2. The diffuse type. This consists of cells with poor cohesion which infiltrate and thicken the stomach wall resulting in the 'linitis plastica' picture. It occurs more commonly in younger people and can develop throughout the stomach, but especially in the cardia.

Other histological types include non-Hodgkin's lymphoma, leiomyosarcoma, squamous carcinomas and carcinoid tumours.

Clinical features

Presentation

Early symptoms include epigastric pain, anorexia, early satiety and weight loss. Nausea and vomiting are frequent, and may be associated with gastric outlet obstruction. Tumours of the oesophago-gastric junction may cause dysphagia. Anaemia from occult blood loss is common, but haematemesis and malaena are more unusual.

Rarely, paraneoplastic syndromes can occur including acanthosis nigricans, dermatomyositis, migratory superficial thrombophlebitis (Trousseau's syndrome), microangiopathic haemolytic anaemia and disseminated intravascular coagulation.

Investigations

Fibreoptic endoscopy. With multiple biopsies and cytological washings this has a diagnostic accuracy approaching 95% in detecting gastric cancer.

Barium meal. With double contrast studies this may also provide best visualization of the tumour. However, false negative rates of up to 25% have been reported and biopsy of the lesion is not possible.

Staging investigations. These should include full blood count, liver function tests and CT scan. Endoscopic ultrasound is being developed and may be more accurate than CT in determining the depth of tumour penetration and the presence of nodal disease.

Staging

Staging of gastric cancer follows the TNM system.

T1	Limited to mucosa or submucosa.
T2	Extension to the serosa.
T3	Penetration through the serosa.
T4	Invasion of adjacent structures.
N0	No nodal involvement.
N1	Local nodal involvement within 3 cm of the primary tumour.
N2	Nodal involvement more than 3 cm from the primary tumour which is resectable.
N3	Distant nodal involvement, which is not resectable.
M0	No distant metastases.
M1	Distant metastases present.

Stage groupings

Stage I:	T1, N0, M.
Stage II:	T2–3, N0, M0.
Stage III:	T1–3, N1–2, M0.
	T4, N0, M0.
Stage IV:	T1–3, N3, M0.
	T4, N1–3, M0.
	any T, any N, M1.

Management

Surgery

Surgical resection is the only curative treatment for gastric carcinoma. The operation is usually either a total or subtotal gastrectomy, along with lymphadenectomy. Splenectomy is not routinely indicated. The extent of the lymphadenectomy is controversial, with Japanese studies showing a survival benefit for extended radical lymphadenectomy.

Surgery can also provide effective palliation in patients with inoperable locally advanced or metastatic disease. Palliative resection of the primary tumour can provide relief from obstruction, bleeding and pain. When resection is not possible, a bypass procedure is sometimes performed.

Radiotherapy

Gastric cancer is relatively resistant to radiotherapy, and complicated by damage to surrounding structures such as the liver, kidneys, small bowel and spinal cord. However, moderate-dose irradiation can be used to palliate symptoms from recurrent or metastatic disease both locally around the stomach bed and at distant sites.

Radiotherapy has been used in an adjuvant setting after potentially curative resection, but so far prospective controlled trials have failed to show a survival benefit. Newer techniques such as intraoperative radiotherapy and combined chemoradiotherapy are being explored.

Chemotherapy

Combination chemotherapy regimens have been reported to produce response rates of up to 45%. The most active single agents include doxorubicin, 5-FU, mitomycin C, cisplatin and the nitrosureas.

More recent drug combinations such as ECF (epirubicin, cisplatin and continuous ambulatory infusion of 5-FU) may have response rates of up to 60%. In advanced disease these regimens are not curative and although moderately toxic, may provide both useful palliation and prolong survival.

The role of both adjuvant and neoadjuvant chemotherapy is under investigation.

Prognostic factors

Gastric cancer presenting early may be amenable to surgical cure, but more than 80% are too advanced for curative resection at the time of presentation. Overall survival is poor, with only 10% of patients alive at 10 years.

Stage of tumour

Stage I:	75%	5 year survival.
Stage II:	30%	5 year survival.
Stage III:	10%	5 year survival.
Stage IV:	2%	5 year survival.

Histology   The diffuse type is associated with a worse prognosis.

Screening

In high-risk populations (e.g. in Japan), mass screening with upper GI endoscopy has increased the early diagnosis and curative surgery rate. However, it is unlikely to be of cost benefit in low-risk populations such as in the UK. An alternative approach would be to screen high-risk groups, such as patients with pernicious anaemia and those who have had previous gastrectomy for benign disease.

Current issues

Development of new surgical techniques, such as extended radical lymphadenectomy, and combining these with adjuvant and neoadjuvant therapies. Specifically, a current MRC trial is evaluating neoadjuvant and adjuvant chemotherapy.

Further reading

Fuchs CS, Mayer RJ. Gastric carcinoma. *New England Journal of Medicine*,1995; **333:** 32–41.

GENE THERAPY

Gene therapy is the treatment of a disease with DNA sequences that encode specific genes. Ideally, gene therapy would specifically replace defective genes with the normal gene *in vivo*. However, the gene transfer technology currently available for clinical use is only able to add genes to cells rather than specifically replace abnormal genes. It may be more useful to modulate immune responses or introduce genes which may modify drug treatments.

The first human gene transfer trial was approved in 1989. The first therapeutic study was used in the treatment of in children with severe combined immune deficiency due to adenosine deaminase (ADA) deficiency. Currently, over 50 clinical gene therapy trials are under way world-wide including the treatment of metabolic deficiencies, cystic fibrosis, HIV and cancer.

Gene transfer technology

Although several studies have used *in vivo* gene transfer, at present this is more frequently performed *in vitro*, with the transduced cells being reintroduced into the patient.

DNA sequences may be delivered to the target cell by physical or viral vectors.

Physical vectors — These include liposomes, polylysine vesicles, calcium phosphate precipitation, gold micro-projectiles and direct micro-injection. Direct injection of DNA into tissues *in vivo* also gives effective gene transfer.

Physical vectors are generally limited by their poor transfection efficiency, that is their ability to transfer DNA sequences to a cell. They do, however, have the advantage of being able to package very large genes.

Viral vectors — These are genetically modified viruses in which pathogenic and replication-associated viral genes are replaced with the gene of interest.

The best characterized vectors are recombinant retroviruses and recombinant adenoviruses. Herpes viruses, adeno-associated viruses and vaccinia viruses are also being developed as gene therapy vectors.

The safety of using viral vectors remains an important issue. Numerous studies using recombinant retroviral vectors and adenoviral vectors are presently in progress.

Targeting therapy — There is a variety of techniques employed to target the therapeutic gene sequences to specific cells:

1. In vitro transfer. The transfer of gene sequences into an isolated population of cells ensures a degree of targeting.

2. In vivo transfer. To target gene therapy to specific cells *in vivo* requires either modification of viral envelopes to target specific cell surface targets for example the EGF receptor, or the incorporation of tissue-specific promoters which precede the transferred gene, for example the tyrosinase promoter to target melanocyte specific gene expression.

Gene therapy approaches

Different strategies have been employed to treat cancer with gene therapy. These include:

Correction of gene defects　This attempts to reverse the malignant phenotype by correcting genetic abnormalities within the cell. Current research is mainly focused on adding normal copies of tumour suppressor genes, for example adding a normal *p53* gene to tumours where this gene is mutated. This approach has been successful in animal studies and has shown clinical effect in a phase one study in human lung cancer (Roth *et al.*, 1996).

Unlike non-malignant disease, such as cystic fibrosis, in which a single gene defect is pathogenic, cancer cells often contain multiple genetic abnormalities. The correction of a single genetic defect may therefore not successfully treat the cancer. Another disadvantage is that only cells that have been successfully transduced will be killed. With the present relatively low efficiency of gene transfer this may only represent a small proportion of cells.

Adding toxic genes　The transfer of genes that encode for cytotoxic proteins has also been considered. At present, however, most approaches transfer a gene that encodes an enzyme that will convert a non-toxic pro-drug into a cytotoxic agent. Examples include transfer of the cytosine deaminase gene that metabolizes the anti-fungal agent 5-fluorocytosine to 5-fluorouracil and the herpes simplex thymidine kinase (*HSVTK*) gene which converts gancyclovir to a toxic metabolite. This system has the advantage of a bystander effect, that is adjacent non-transduced dividing cells are also killed, thus obviating the need for all cells to be transduced. *HSVTK* gene transfer using retroviral and adenoviral is currently being used in clinical trials.

Immunomodulation

Many of the current gene therapy studies have focused on trying to enhance the immune response. This reduces the need to target all cells with the gene transfer as an activated immune response may be able to detect and kill non-transfected tumour cells. Gene transfer of immuno-stimulatory cytokine genes, for example *IL-2*, *GM-CSF* and *TNF*, into tumour cells is being evaluated in human trials. In animal models, tumour cells engineered to secrete cytokines can be used as therapeutic 'vaccines' to treat established tumours.

Vaccination by gene transfer of tumour antigen genes is effective in animal models and is presently being evaluated in clinical studies, for example the human papilloma virus *E6* gene in cervical carcinoma.

Current issues

The initial clinical studies with gene transfer have essentially monitored safety and feasibility, and have demonstrated that this approach is possible. Results of their efficacy are awaited. Current research is aimed at improving gene transfer efficiency and targeting by development of new vectors. This will increase the number of possible approaches and the genes that may be suitable for transfer.

Further reading

Roth UH *et al.* Retrovirus mediated wild-type *p53* gene transfer to tumours of patients with lung cancer. *Nature Medicine*, 1996; 985–91.

Related topic of interest

Molecular biology of cancer (p. 151)

HEAD AND NECK CANCER

Head and neck cancer refers to tumours originating in the oral cavity, pharynx, larynx and paranasal sinuses.

Background

Incidence

Head and neck tumours comprise approximately 4% of all tumours in the UK, with about 2000 new cases and 900 deaths per year. The most common anatomical site is the larynx, representing about 2–3% of all malignant disease and more than 80% of head and neck cancer.

Risk factors

The main risk factors in the UK are tobacco and alcohol use. World-wide, tobacco or betel nut chewing and the incidence of Epstein–Barr virus infection are important in certain malignancies.

Aetiology

The molecular pathogenesis of head and neck cancer remains ill-defined. Chromosome deletions in the region of p16 (9p21), a cyclin-dependent kinase inhibitor, suggest this may act as a tumour-suppressor gene. The *p53* gene is also frequently mutated.

Histology

Ninety per cent of head and neck cancers are squamous cell in origin. The remainder are almost all adenocarcinoma. Lymphoma is uncommon, and head and neck melanoma rare.

Spread is mainly to regional lymph nodes, with spread commonly occurring before a lump is palpable. Early haematogenous spread is rare (to lung and bone when it does occur).

Head and neck cancer frequently presents with more than one primary tumour. This is believed to represent a field change within the epithelial tissues of the head and neck following carcinogenic exposure.

Clinical features

Presentation

The anatomical diversity of head and neck cancer leads to a wide spectrum of clinical presentation. It may also determine the stage at which a disease presents. Tumours producing obvious symptoms (hoarse voice in laryngeal cancer, difficulties with chewing, swallowing or speaking in carcinoma of the tongue) tend to present early. Carcinoma of the hypopharynx generally presents late with dysphagia. Many oropharyngeal malignancies are detected at routine dental review.

Facial nerve palsies associated with swelling of the parotid salivary gland should always be suspected of being due to malignant rather than benign disease.

Investigations

Indirect laryngoscopy/nasendoscopy may visualize the tumour, but examination under anaesthetic with biopsy is preferable for optimal imaging and tissue diagnosis. Fine-needle aspiration of involved lymph nodes may also achieve a cytological diagnosis.

CT is required for assessment of lymph node involvement.

Staging

The TNM system defines the staging for all head and neck cancers.

Management

Management of head and neck cancer frequently requires a multi-disciplinary approach. The mainstays of management are surgery and/or radiotherapy. Initial assessment therefore frequently takes place in a combined ENT/Radiotherapy clinic.

Allied professionals such as speech therapists and dieticians, are invaluable in the management of speech and swallowing difficulties which may result from the effects of the tumour or its treatment.

Surgery

Radical surgical techniques may be used to achieve long-term survival or cure. Resection of the primary tumour with associated lymph nodes frequently requires major reconstruction. The role of more selective surgery with limited resection of local tissue and lymph nodes is under investigation.

Radiotherapy

Radiotherapy may be given as the primary curative treatment for certain tumours, for example T1 or T2 tumours of the larynx. Radiotherapy is also the treatment of choice in nasopharyngeal carcinoma and oropharyngeal cancer, where surgery may cause problems with the flow of air or nutrients. Radiotherapy may also be employed for relapse after surgery and as an adjuvant to primary surgical therapy.

External beam radiotherapy is most frequently employed. However, the use of brachytherapy, involving implantation of iridium wires, caesium needles, gold grains or radium moulds, can be particularly useful in tumours such as those involving the tongue.

Chemotherapy

Chemotherapy has generally been used in patients with metastatic or locally recurrent disease. Combination chemotherapy with drugs such as such as cisplatin, 5-fluorouracil, methotrexate or doxorubicin may achieve response rates of up to 50%. These responses are generally short-lived and not associated with improved survival.

The role of chemotherapy in combination therapy with surgery and/or radiotherapy is the focus of current trials. New agents such as the taxanes and gemcitabine are under investigation.

Prognostic factors

Stage of tumour

The stage of disease at presentation, determined to some extent by the site of the primary tumour, is the most powerful prognostic indicator.

Site of tumour

1. *Laryngeal.* T1 and T2 tumours are almost always curable by radiotherapy.

2. *Tongue.* Tumours of the tip of the tongue are much easier to control than the lateral margins.

3. *Oral cavity.* T1/T2 and T4 oral cavity tumours have 5-year overall survival figures of 60–90% and less than 30%, respectively.

4. *Oropharynx.* Survival is generally poor: 10–15% 5 year survival.

Related topic of interest

Cell cycle (p. 40)

HEPATOCELLULAR CARCINOMA

Primary liver tumours are rare in the UK. However, in the developing world, especially the Far East and Africa, hepatocellular carcinoma (HCC or hepatoma) is one of the most prevalent cancers.

Background

Incidence

In the UK there are approximately 1500 new cases per year, occurring predominantly in 40–60 year olds. In endemic areas of the world, its incidence approaches 100 per 100 000 of the population and occurs mainly in the 20–40 age group. World-wide, the male to female ratio is 3:2, but this male predominance is more marked (11:1) in cases where liver cirrhosis is the pathogenic mechanism.

Aetiology

World-wide, the two major aetiological agents are micro-organisms. Hepatocellular carcinoma therefore represents a potentially preventable tumour.

1. Hepatitis B virus. There is a close correlation between the geographical distribution of the cancer, and the prevalence of the virus. Double-stranded DNA viral genome is detectable in 80% of cases of HCC in endemic areas, with a relative risk of 230:1.

2. Aflatoxin. This is present in stored cereals contaminated with the mould Aspergillus flavus.

3. Liver cirrhosis. The most common cause in Western society is liver cirrhosis of any cause, for example alcohol, haemochromatosis and primary biliary cirrhosis (PBC). However, even in the UK, HCC is rare in alcoholic cirrhotic patients who are seronegative for the hepatitis B virus (HBV) surface antigen.

4. Non-cirrhotic causes. These include some forms of radiological contrast medium and androgenic anabolic steroids.

Histology	HCC is the most common primary hepatic malignancy. Cholangiocarcinoma and hepatic angiosarcoma occur less frequently. Hepatoblastoma is a rare tumour of childhood.
	HCC usually arises either from the liver parenchyma or a cirrhotic nodule. In 60% of cases, the tumour is multi-focal, 30% are solitary lesions, and the remaining 10% involve diffuse infiltration of the tumour. They are usually fast-growing and large at presentation. Most stain positively with antibody against α-fetoprotein (AFP).

Clinical features

Presentation	Presenting symptoms and signs are frequently due to direct tumour effects, such as right upper quadrant pain, or to associated complications, such as venous thromboses or IVC compression. HCC may also present with symptoms attributable to non-metastatic manifestations of the tumour, including ectopic production of a variety of hormones.
Investigations	Liver function tests, including prothrombin time are often deranged in HCC, but are not sufficiently specific to be diagnostically useful. In 90% of cases serum AFP is raised.
	Radiological investigations in HCC include liver ultrasound and/or CT scanning. Chest CT to detect pulmonary metastases is required if liver transplantation is contemplated. Angiography is only required if assessment of the vascular supply of the tumour is necessary prior to surgery or tumour embolization.
	Biopsy of the tumour may be either percutaneous under radiological guidance, or direct at laparotomy or laparoscopy.
Staging	There is no staging system in routine clinical use.

Management

Surgery is the only potentially curative therapy in cases of HCC that have already arisen. However, in endemic areas, where two of the major pathogenic mechanisms involve micro-organisms, preventative medicine may be of value in reducing morbidity and mortality.

Prevention	Preventative measures include HBV vaccination and health education regarding the modes of spread of the virus, and improved storage of cereals prone to *Aspergillus* colonization.
Surgery	Curative surgery may involve either hepatic lobectomy or complete liver transplant. Cirrhotic patients are prone to decompensating their liver disease peri-operatively, necessitating careful patient selection. Only 5–10% are suitable for such surgery.
	Palliative surgery includes ligation of the hepatic artery to reduce the nutritive supply to the growing tumour. This treatment, associated with a 5% mortality, is often of short-lived benefit, as collateral blood supplies rapidly develop. Following angiographic embolization of the hepatic artery, collaterals develop more slowly. The process can be repeated in cases of relapse.
Radiotherapy	HCC is not highly radio-sensitive. However, palliative radiotherapy can produce symptomatic relief of capsular pain.
Chemotherapy	Chemotherapy does not have a major role in palliative management of HCC, though good response rates can be achieved with doxorubicin or etoposide. Locally targeted chemotherapy, via intra-hepatic arterial administration, is currently under trial.

Prognostic factors

The prognosis for HCC is poor. Untreated cases almost all die within 1 year. Cirrhotic patients have a median survival of 3 months, and zero at 1 year. Non-cirrhotic patients have a 10% 2 year overall survival. Even in carefully selected patients treated with resection or transplantation, 5 year disease-free survival is in the order of 15–20%, though this can rise to 50% in those with tumours less than 3 cm at resection.

Screening

In the developed world, screening of high-risk patients (for example those with known causes of cirrhosis such as haemochromatosis) using serum AFP levels may allow early detection of tumour development via rising AFP levels, permitting early intervention.

Current issues

The ability of intra-hepatic arterial chemotherapy to improve response rates is a focus of current research.

HODGKIN'S DISEASE

Hodgkin's disease is a lymphoid malignancy. Over the last 30 years it has become curable for many patients.

Background

Incidence

In Western Europe the incidence is 2–3 per 100 000 population but this varies world-wide. In the UK approximately 1500 cases are diagnosed each year, with a male to female ratio of 3:2. There are two incidence peaks, at 20–25 and after 50 years.

Aetiology

Siblings of young patients have a seven-fold increased risk that might be genetic or environmental. The Epstein–Barr virus (EBV) has been implicated as a causative agent with histological similarities between the lymph nodes of Hodgkin's and EBV patients. EBV may simply alter host immunity as the incidence is higher in the immunosuppressed.

Histology

The diagnosis is histological, based on tissue containing characteristic malignant cells (mononuclear Hodgkin's cells or multinucleated Reed–Sternberg cells) in an appropriate multicellular stroma. Stains for immunological surface markers help diagnosis. The histology has some correlation with epidemiology, stage at presentation, and hence prognosis which led to subclassification via the Rye classification.

1. Nodular sclerosis. This is the most common, particularly in young patients and with limited supradiaphragmatic disease representing 75% of cases. It often has a better prognosis, although this probably depends on the cellular content of the nodules.

2. Lymphocyte-predominant. This is often nodular in pattern and has a strongly lymphocytic stroma with fewer malignant cells. It is rare and tends to present with early stage disease, peripheral nodes, and an indolent course with late relapses.

3. *Lymphocyte-depleted.* This has few lymphocytes and more malignant cells. It is the least common, presents in older patients usually with more advanced disease and poor outlook and may not have always been easily differentiated from NHL.

4. *Mixed cellularity.* In this the stroma contains many different cell lines. It makes up one quarter of cases, particularly with sub-diaphragmatic disease. Prognosis is intermediate.

Clinical features

Presentation

Most patients present with painless lymphadenopathy, most often cervical. Extranodal disease occurs in less than 15%. Fever, drenching night sweats, or unexplained 10% weight loss occur in 30% of patients are defined as 'B' symptoms and affect the staging of the patient (see below). Patients without B symptoms are defined as stage A. Itching and alcohol-induced pains are also recognized.

Investigations

The aims are tissue diagnosis, prognostic staging, detecting complications, and guiding treatment.

A tissue diagnosis should be made in every case following examination of an adequate biopsy.

The sites and bulk of disease are determined by CT scanning of the chest, abdomen and pelvis. The nodes involved are usually contiguous. The treatment of Hodgkin's is highly dependent on stage (see below) and therefore equivocally enlarged nodes should be biopsied. B symptoms, anaemia and elevated erythrocyte sedimentation rate or lactate dehydrogenase suggest bulky disease.

Full blood count, urea and electrolytes, and liver biochemistry can detect complications and influence treatment. Patients with extensive disease, or unexplained abnormal haematology, need bone marrow assessment.

Staging laparotomy has been extensively used and may alter the stage compared with CT in many patients. It has not been shown to alter survival and is used now in the UK very rarely.

| Staging | This is based upon the system formalized at Ann Arbor in 1971 but developed at the Cotswold meeting in 1989. |

Stage I: Involvement of a single lymph node region or a lymphoid structure.

Stage II: Two or more lymph node regions or structures on one side of the diaphragm. A suffix number denotes the number of sites of disease.

Stage III: Involvement of lymph node regions or structures on both sides of the diaphragm.

Stage IV: Disseminated involvement of extralymphatic organs with or without lymph nodes.

Patients are subclassified as A or B depending upon the presence of 'B' symptoms.

Management

Surgery

As Hodgkin's disease is such a radio- and chemo-sensitive disease surgical resection is not required.

Radiotherapy

Small volume, good prognosis stage 1 and 2A disease can be treated with radiotherapy. Radiotherapy fields are often extended to include contiguous nodes as these are often the site of relapse (e.g. the extended 'mantle' for cervical disease and the 'inverted Y' field for inguinal disease). For such early stage disease, overall prognosis is unaffected if relapse is treated with chemotherapy. The addition of chemotherapy to radiotherapy in all patients with early stage disease is therefore not justified.

Sites of bulky disease in higher stage patients may be irradiated following initial chemotherapy.

Chemotherapy

Combination chemotherapy forms the basis of treatment for patients with stage 2B or greater disease. The regimens most commonly used in the UK are ChlVPP (chlorambucil/vinblastine/procarbazine/prednisolone), and ABVD (adriamycin/bleomycin/vinblastine/dacarbazine) or related regimens where dacarbazine is replaced by etoposide (e.g. PABLOE). Standard treatment is alternating regimens of ChlVPP with either PABLOE or ABVD.

Hodgkin's disease is one of the few solid tumours in which high-dose chemotherapy has been shown, in randomized trials, to be of benefit to selected patients. Patients who relapse after standard chemotherapy may be treated with high-dose BEAM (carmustine/etoposide/cytarabine/melphalan) or CBV (cyclophosphamide/carmustine/etoposide) and supported with blood stem cell rescue. There may also be a role for high-dose treatments in the initial therapy of a proportion of patients who present with advanced disease, although defining this poor risk group is difficult.

For young patients, who have such an excellent prognosis, future fertility should be considered. 'Sperm banking' should be offered. In the future the cryopreservation of ovarian sections may be possible.

Prognostic factors

The major prognostic indicators are histological type, grade, stage, number of involved sites, bulk of disease, age, performance status and LDH.

For patients with small volume stage 1 and 2 disease, the cure rate is 80%. With more extensive disease, 50% of patients are cured using combination chemotherapy. All patients who relapse should be considered for further chemotherapy, as a significant proportion of these (30–40%) may still be cured.

Current issues

Current therapy is highly effective. The focus of many current trials is therefore to assess the ability to reduce late toxicity such as infertility, secondary malignancy and cardiomyopathy, by reducing the amount of treatment.

Further reading

Yeun AR, Horning SJ. Recent advances in Hodgkin's disease. *Current Opinion in Haematology*, **4:** 286–90.

HYPERCALCAEMIA

Hypercalcaemia occurs in 10–20% of cancer patients and may be associated with significant morbidity. Treating hypercalcaemia can significantly improve symptoms and quality of life. ־

Causes

In patients with cancer, hypercalcaemia is most frequently due to the malignancy. However, other non-malignant causes should be considered, for example hyperparathyroidism or drugs.

Malignant hypercalcaemia is associated with carcinoma of the breast (20–40% of malignancy-induced hypercalcaemia), lung (25–35%), kidney and haematological malignancies (multiple myeloma).

Aetiology

Malignant hypercalcaemia may result from diverse aetiological processes and does not imply the presence of advanced metastatic disease. It may result from:

1. Increased bone resorption. Mobilization of calcium may result from direct bone destruction (osteolysis) by bony metastases or primary bone tumour.

Indirect bone resorption may be induced by circulating factors produced by tumours. This is most frequently seen with breast and squamous cell lung cancers. Parathyroid-like hormones [parathyroid hormone related peptide (PTHRP)] and other growth factors, such as TNF, TGF-α and TGF-β, have been implicated. These predominantly act via increased osteoclast activity.

2. Decreased calcium excretion. A reduction in renal clearance of calcium may result from renal disease (e.g. myeloma kidney) or the effects of the circulating factors.

3. Associated factors. Hypercalcaemia of malignancy may be potentiated by immobility, concurrent drug therapy (such as oestrogens and thiazide diuretics) and conditions that reduce renal excretion.

Clinical features

Presentation

The symptoms of hypercalcaemia are usually non-specific and include drowsiness, confusion, nausea, vomiting and polyuria leading to dehydration. The severity of symptoms often does not correlate with the serum calcium level. Many patients remain asymptomatic.

Management

Treatment

There are three aims of treatment:

1. Symptomatic treatment. The initial treatment involves correcting volume depletion with 2–3 litres or more in the first 24 hours.

2. Specific hypocalcaemic treatment

- Bisphosphonates are potent inhibitors of osteoclasts, binding hydroxyapatite in calcified bone and thereby preventing bone resorption. IV Pamidronate is currently standard first-line therapy and is effective in approximately 80% of cases. Oral preparations of bisphosphonates can be given for maintenance therapy. Bisphosphonates take 3–4 days to work and the effects usually last for 7 to 30 days.
- Mithramycin is an inhibitor of osteoclast RNA synthesis which has now largely been replaced by the bisphosphonates because of its toxicity (bone marrow suppression, liver and kidney toxicity). However, its calcium-lowering effects are generally quicker than the biphosphonates.
- Steroids can also lower the calcium level, but are rarely helpful in the management of malignant hypercalcaemia. Their main use is in steroid-responsive tumours, such as lymphoma. Their mode of action is thought to be by a combination of increasing urinary calcium excretion, inhibiting osteoclast activity and decreasing GI absorption.

- For more resistant cases, alternatives include calcitonin, octreotide and oral phosphate therapy. Frusemide will lower the calcium level by inhibiting renal tubular calcium reabsorption, but needs to be carefully administered with adequate fluid replacement.

3. Treatment of the underlying diagnosis. Effective treatment of the underlying malignancy is the most reliable method of reducing a malignant hypercalcaemia in the long term. However, in many cases treatment of the hypercalcaemia is palliative.

Current issues

New drugs

Newer bisphosphonates, such as ibandronate, are being developed, and trials are in progress. Its advantage is that it can be given as bolus injection and the efficacy is greater.

Related topic of interest

Multiple myeloma (p. 160)
Paraneoplastic syndromes (p. 201)

IMMUNOTHERAPY

Immunotherapy for cancer has been attempted for over a century, with only limited success to date. The basis for immunotherapy is the recognition that the host defences can play a role in tumour identification and elimination.

Background

The immune system consists of several effector cells that can recognize and kill tumour cells. These include the following.

B cells B cells produce antibodies that recognize foreign and abnormal soluble secreted proteins or cell-surface proteins. Although binding of antibody to such antigens can induce antibody-directed cell cytotoxicity (ADCC), antibodies are predominantly responsible for destroying extracellular pathogens and are usually thought to play a less important role in cell killing.

T cells T lymphocytes play a central role in the recognition and elimination of abnormal cells. Two main subtypes exist:

- T-helper lymphocytes: secrete cytokines (soluble messenger proteins), which co-ordinate the immune response.
- Cytotoxic T lymphocytes (CTLs): kill target cells.

T cells recognize abnormal cells by binding of the T-cell receptor with peptides (derived from processed antigens) presented within the groove of the HLA molecules on the target cell. This gives a mechanism where any cell making abnormal intracellular proteins could potentially be detected and killed by T cells. This applies to virally infected cells that produce foreign, viral proteins or tumour cells making mutated proteins. Tumour-specific antigens have now been identified that can be recognized by CTLs.

NK cells Natural killer cells (NK cells) are lymphocytes that can kill virally infected or tumour cells, although the precise recognition elements that they use are not defined. NK cells do not need prior exposure to an antigen to be able to mount a response. If lymphocytes are grown *in vitro* in a high concentration of IL-2, a lymphocyte growth factor, a population of lymphokine-activated killer (LAK) cells which have similar but broader activity can be obtained.

Macrophages　　Macrophages are also potent killers of tumour cells, but again the precise recognition elements are not defined.

Antigen presentation

To elicit an effective immune response, these cells need to receive appropriate 'costimulatory signals' as well as recognizing foreign or abnormal proteins or else a state of anergy (tolerance) develops. Macrophages and dendritic cells can provide these co-stimulatory signals via cell-surface proteins (e.g. the B7 molecule) and play a major role in antigen presentation. Once activated, numerous cytokines (including IL-2, IFNγ, TNF) are produced which enhance and modulate the immune response.

Tumour antigens

Antigens are proteins that can elicit a specific antibody or a T-cell response and can be tumour specific, being present only on or in tumour cells (tumour specific antigens, TSAs). More commonly they are tumour associated, being present on some normal tissues but overexpressed on tumour cells (e.g. GM2, cERB-2, tyrosinase).

Several tumour antigens recognized by antibodies exist. More recently antigens recognized by T cells have also been isolated. These include the MAGE family of antigens, which encode proteins normally only made in the testis, but which are overexpressed in many tumours. Other such antigens that can induce a T-cell response include the tyrosinase protein found in normal and malignant melanocytes and the E7 protein of the human papilloma virus found in cervical cancer.

Immunotherapy

Immunotherapy aims to enhance the body's natural response to foreign or mutated proteins to cause effective elimination of the tumour by active or passive mechanisms.

Passive　　Involves administration of effectors generated *in vitro* [e.g. monoclonal antibodies or LAK cells (also called adoptive immunotherapy)]. Attempts can be made to modify these to make them more effective (e.g. by conjugating toxins or radioactive isotopes to antibodies). To date passive immunotherapy has not generally been successful. Encouraging results have been seen with antibodies to B cell lymphomas (ante CD19 and CD20) and some colonic cancer antibodies.

Active

Aims at inducing activation of the host immune response either by vaccination or by administering cytokines.

1. Vaccination with a variety of antigen preparations has been tried for numerous tumours.

- Non-specific: aimed at general immune activation (e.g. with BCG). This approach has been very successful in the treatment of *in situ* carcinoma of the bladder. Its use mainly as an adjuvant in the treatment of other cancers has however been disappointing.
- Specific: aims to activate antigen-specific immune responses by vaccination with antigen. Whole cells, crude cell membrane extracts, purified proteins and peptides are all being investigated. These are often given with a non-specific immunogen (an adjuvant) which probably acts by enhancing antigen presentation and co-stimulation. To date few have been proven to warrant generalized use. Encouraging preliminary data have been seen in the treatment of melanoma with a three-melanoma cell line vaccine, and with vaccination of the GM2 ganglioside (a membrane protein overexpressed on melanoma cells).

2. Cytokines. Administration of cytokines has been attempted to enhance the host immune response. The most widely used are IFN-α and IL-2. Some modest but consistent responses have been seen, in some cancers notably renal carcinoma and melanoma. There are occasionally long-term remissions.

Current issues

Gene therapy

With the delineation of novel tumour antigens and the molecular mechanisms of the anti-tumour response there has been much interest in using gene therapy to enhance the immune response. Transfer of genes encoding cytokines or co-stimulatory molecules into tumours or lymphocytes have been successful in animal models and are being investigated in human trials.

Vaccines	Novel vaccination approaches using dendritic cells or peptide antigens are currently being developed.
Cytokines	New cytokines currently being investigated in the clinic and in the laboratory for their immune anti-tumour effects include IL-7, IL-12, IL-15 and IL-18.

Further reading

DeVita VT, Hellman S, Rosenberg SA. *Biological Therapy of Cancer*, JB Lippincott, 1995.

Related topics of interest

Biological therapy (p. 7)
Interleukin-2 (p. 123)
Melanoma – malignant (p. 143)

INTERLEUKIN-2

Interleukin-2 (IL-2) is a cytokine secreted by T lymphocytes that causes activation and proliferation of several effector cells of the immune system. The purified protein is available in quantities suitable for administration into humans as an immunotherapeutic agent.

Uses

IL-2 at present only has a licence for use in the treatment of metastatic renal cancer. The response rate as a single agent is approximately 15%. Its anti-tumour effect has been evaluated in several other tumour types such as malignant melanoma. The response rate in advanced melanoma is approximately 20%. Higher response rates have been seen with combinations of chemotherapy, interferon and IL-2. Occasional long-term survival is achieved following IL-2 treatment.

Mode of action

IL-2 exerts its actions by binding to the IL-2 receptor, which is present on activated T lymphocytes, B lymphocytes, NK cells and macrophages. This initiates a series of changes leading to proliferation of these effectors and to their further differentiation. Cytotoxic T lymphocytes become further activated with increased cytotoxicity and secretion of secondary cytokines such as TNF and IFN-γ. IL-2 also causes increased cytotoxicity and cytokine release from NK cells and macrophages. It is this immune activation that is predominantly responsible for the *in vitro* and *in vivo* anti-tumour effects of IL-2.

Pharmacokinetics

IL-2 has a very short half-life in the circulation (approximately 10 min). At the doses used in treatment is thought to be in part protein bound, in particular being bound by soluble IL-2 receptors. The exact means of elimination is unclear, although thought to be mainly degraded by the kidney.

Scheduling

The optimal mode of administration is still unclear. Several have been investigated including the following.

1. High-dose IV bolus. Used more commonly in the USA. Approximately 6×10^5 units/kg given over 15 minutes three times a day, for 4–6 days, every 2–3 weeks. This is associated with marked toxicity often requiring intensive care.

2. Intermediate-dose continuous infusion. Used more in Europe. Approximately 18×10^6 units/m²/day for 3–5 days. Overall approximately one third of the total dose achievable by bolus administration can be given with markedly reduced toxicity although hospital admission is required.

3. Subcutaneous bolus. Doses of approximately 10–20 U/m²/day. Toxicity is less than with IV administration but it remains to be seen whether it is as effective.

Toxicity

- Capillary leak syndrome. IL-2 can cause an acute 'leakiness' of capillaries by an unknown mechanism. This leads to pulmonary oedema, cerebral oedema, intravascular fluid depletion and hence weight gain, hypotension and ultimately oliguric renal failure. IV fluids and inotropic support may enable the IL-2 infusion to continue.
- Cardiac arrhythmias.
- Confusion and in severe cases coma. This is more common with high-dose IV boluses.
- Infections. Patients can behave as if immunosuppressed and are particularly prone to bacterial infections.
- Nausea and vomiting can be quite severe, requiring ondansetron.
- Fever and rigors are very common as with most cytokines.
- Local reactions. Local inflammation is seen at subcutaneous injection sites.
- Autoimmune disease, in particular hypothyroidism.

Current issues

The role of IL-2 in the treatment of renal cancer and melanoma is still unclear. Present studies are investigating the use of combination chemotherapy with immunotherapies. Strategies for achieving local IL-2 secretion by gene therapy are being investigated.

Further reading

Atkins MB, Mier JW. *Therapeutic Applications of Interleukin-2.* Marcel Dekker, 1993.

Related topics of interest

Biological therapy (p. 7)
Immunotherapy (p. 119)
Melanoma – malignant (p. 143)

LEUKAEMIA – ACUTE

Background

Incidence

Almost 6000 cases of acute leukaemia are diagnosed in adults each year in the UK. Approximately 80% are acute myeloblastic leukaemia (AML), while 20% are acute lymphoblastic leukaemia (ALL). ALL is the most common leukaemia of childhood.

Aetiology

Acute leukaemia is believed to result from neoplastic transformation of a single haemopoietic precursor. This malignant change leads to an inappropriate clonal proliferation of cells unable to undergo full differentiation into the mature phenotype.

The precise nature of genetic abnormalities associated with leukaemogenesis are under investigation. Chromosomal translocations are frequent and produce functional proteins with inappropriate control of expression. Single gene mutations such as *ras* and *p53* have been identified in both AML and ALL.

Risk factors

A variety of factors have been identified which are associated with an increased of acute leukaemia. These include:

1. *Congenital disorders.* These include, for example Down's syndrome and Kleinfelter's syndrome.

2. *Ionizing radiation.* A 20-fold increase in acute leukaemia occurred following the Hiroshima atomic bomb. The clustering of childhood leukaemia around the Sellafield has been attributed to radiation experienced by the father prior to conception (Gardner *et al.*, 1990).

3. *Chemical exposure.* Chemotherapy exposure, especially alkylating agents, is associated with AML in particular.

4. *Infective agent.* The role of an infective agent in childhood leukaemia remains controversial.

Histology

The acute leukaemias are classified as myeloblastic (arising from myeloid progenitors) and lymphoblastic (arising from lymphoid progenitors). Cytochemical, immunological and cytogenetic analyses help to make the diagnosis in difficult cases. They are further subdivided by the French–American classification (FAB).

1. AML

MO   Undifferentiated myeloblastic leukaemia.
M1   Myeloblastic leukaemia without maturation.
M2   Myeloblastic leukaemia with maturation.
M3   Promyelocytic leukaemia.
M4   Myelomonocytic leukaemia.
M5   Monocytic/monoblastic leukaemia.
M6   Erythroleukaemia.
M7   Megakaryoblastic leukaemia.

2. ALL

L1   Small blasts, scanty cytoplasm, high nuclear-to-cytoplasmic ratio.
L2   Larger blasts, more cytoplasm, heterogenous in size and shape.
L3   Large blasts with basophilic cytoplasm.

Immunophenotyping performed on the basis of expression of surface molecules defines ALL as B-cell lineage, T-cell lineage or null-cell lineage.

Clinical features

Presentation

Patients present with the clinical consequences of bone marrow failure: infections, anaemia, bruising and bleeding or non-specific complaints of tiredness or lethargy. Bone pain is common. At the time of diagnosis there may be evidence of leukaemic infiltration of other organs, for example hepatosplenomegaly, lymphadenopathy, gum hypertrophy, meningeal involvement and testicular enlargement. Very high white-cell counts can lead to hyperviscosity syndrome with headaches, drowsiness and confusion, progressing into fits and focal neurological signs.

Investigations

Peripheral blood. White-cell counts may be reduced or normal in 40% of patients. White-cell counts greater than 50 x $10^9/l$ occur more frequently in ALL. Anaemia and thrombocytopenia frequently occur. Coagulation abnormalities are frequent and are classically associated with promyelocytic AML (M3).

Bone marrow aspirate. This is essential to confirm a diagnosis of leukaemia and allows accurate sub-typing of the disease with immunophenotyping and cytogenetics.

Lumbar puncture. This is used to exclude CNS involvement.

CXR. T-ALL in particular may present with lymphadenopathy especially of the mediastinum.

Management

Supportive

Following diagnosis, prompt treatment of the infective, haematological and metabolic complications associated with acute leukaemia is essential. Such management is essential for the duration of the patient's treatment.

1. Infection. The absolute or functional neutropenia induced by either the disease or its treatment means that prompt management of infection is essential. Broad-spectrum antibiotics should be commenced immediately prior to confirmation with cultures. These patients are at a high risk of picking up atypical infection. Aspergillus, Pneumocystis *carinii* and viruses can cause life-threatening infections in the patients.

2. Haematological. Bleeding may be due to a deficiency in platelets (numbers or functional capacity) or clotting factors. Platelet or plasma infusions are given as appropriate to treat, or ideally prevent, bleeding. Disseminated intravascular coagulation (DIC) occurs frequently with promyelocytic leukaemia and is best treated with specific anti-leukaemia treatment.

3. Metabolic. Initial induction therapy may precipitate tumour lysis syndrome (raised potassium and uric acid, urate nephropathy). The administration of allopurinol and maintenance of a good diuresis help avoid this.

Chemotherapy

Leukaemia is extremely sensitive to combination chemotherapy. Complete response to initial induction therapy is between 60% and 90% for ALL and approximately 65% for AML. Following the induction of complete remission, considerable disease may still be present which may rapidly lead to relapse. Post-remission therapy is therefore used in attempt to eradicate this sub-clinical disease.

1. Induction. AML is frequently treated with a combination of daunorubicin and cytarabine. The addition of additional drugs, such as etoposide or mitozantrone, is under investigation. ALL induction therapy includes prednisolone, vincristine and anthracyclines. Additional drugs, such as cyclophosphamide or asparaginase, may be used.

CNS disease may be treated with intrathecal cytarabine or methotrexate.

Promyelocytic leukaemia, with characteristic cytogenetics (t(15:17) translocation), may be treated to remission with all-*trans* retinoic acid (ATRA). ATRA induces differentiation of the malignant clone and induces a complete remission in 70–90% of patients.

2. Post-remission. In AML this may be given as 'consolidation' (short-term, relatively intensive, cytarabine-based chemotherapy similar to induction) or 'intensification' (dose-intensive, cytarabine-based treatment or high-dose marrow-ablative chemotherapy with bone marrow rescue). Both of these approaches are more effective than 'maintenance' (longer term, low-dose chemotherapy).

ALL post-remission therapy may be given as high-dose marrow-ablative chemotherapy with bone marrow support or 'intensification' followed by 'maintenance' therapy.

	Treatment with high-dose chemotherapy and bone marrow transplant is generally equivalent to that achieved with other regimes. This is due to the morbidity and mortality associated with the procedure, for example graft-versus-host disease (GVHD) and interstitial pneumonitis.
Radiotherapy	Radiotherapy is often combined with chemotherapy as part of a marrow ablative regime pre-bone marrow transplant. It may also be effective in treating symptomatic areas of leukaemic infiltration.
	Cranial irradiation can be used for CNS disease.

Prognostic factors

Sixty to eighty per cent of patients achieve complete remission after induction therapy, with a median duration of remission of 15 months. Relapse after remission is generally fatal within a year, even if a second remission can be achieved.

Adverse prognostic features include older age group, male sex, white-cell count over $30 \times 10^9/l$ at the time of diagnosis, CNS involvement, certain cytogenetic abnormalities, and more than 4 weeks taken to achieve a complete remission.

The prognosis for childhood leukaemia has improved significantly over the last 20 years, with a 5-year survival rate of 65–75%. Unfortunately, the same cannot be said for adult disease whose survival at 5 years is only 20–35%. AML sufferers have a better prognosis: 40–60% 5 year survival for those aged below 55 and 20% for those over 55 years of age.

Further reading

Gardner MJ *et al.* Results of case-centred study of leukaemia and lymphoma among young people near Sellafield nuclear plant in West Cumbria. *British Medical Journal*, 1990; **300:** 423–9.

Lesner RJ, Goldstone AH. ABC of clinical haematology: the acute leukaemias. *British Medical Journal*, 1997; **314:** 733–6.

Related topic of interest

Leukaemia – chronic (p. 131)

LEUKAEMIA – CHRONIC

Chronic myeloid leukaemia (CML) and chronic lymphocytic leukaemia (CLL) develop from neoplastic proliferation of a white-cell precursor cell. In both conditions the neoplastic clone retains some ability to differentiate towards the mature cell. The 'chronic' nature of the conditions refers to the disease's natural comparison with the acute leukamias.

Chronic myeloid leukaemia

CML is one of a group of disorders known as the myeloproliferative disorders. These include polycythaemia, essential thromobocythaemia and myelofibrosis.

Incidence

CML accounts for 15% of all leukaemias with approximately 700 new cases in the UK each year. The average age of onset is 40–45 years but the disease may affect any age. Males are affected slightly more than females with a ratio of 1.4:1.

Risk factors

Clustering of cases occurred after the atomic bomb and also in patients who received radiotherapy for ankylosing spondylitis.

Aetiology

The Philadelphia chromosome is the characteristic cytogenetic finding in CML. This abnormality results from a translocation between chromosomes 9 and 22. This translocation results in the synthesis of a protein which has tyrosine kinase activity and thus enables the leukaemic clone to resist apoptosis (programmed cell death). Over 95% of patients are Philadelphia chromosome positive.

Histology

Increased numbers of white cells (generally between $100 \times 10^9/l$ and $300 \times 10^9/l$) are found in peripheral blood, with normal numbers of lymphocytes. The bone marrow is generally hypercellular with an increase in the myeloid progenitor cells, megakaryocytes and other white cell lineages (basophils, eosinophils).

Clinical features

Presentation

20% of patients are asymptomatic at diagnosis with the disease found on routine blood tests. Symptoms may include fatigue, weight loss, fever, sweats, bruising and, uncommonly, those related to a hyperviscosity syndrome (e.g. headaches and visual disturbance). The patient may complain of abdominal distension or pain secondary to splenic or hepatic enlargement or infarction. Lymphadenopathy may be present. Patients may present with gout.

Investigations

FBC. The diagnosis can be made from a blood test. The white-cell count is raised with an excess of neutrophils, basophils and eosinophils; blasts may be present. The haemoglobin may be reduced and the platelet count elevated.

Bone-marrow aspirate/trephine. The diagnosis of CML can be made on a peripheral blood film, but most clinicians perform a bone-marrow examination to confirm the diagnosis.

Neutrophil alkaline phosphatase. The score is typically low, excluding a reactive neutrophilia.

Vitamin B_{12} and B_{12}-binding capacity. This is typically elevated in CML.

Cytogenetic study of the bone marrow. This reveals the presence of the Philadelphia chromosome.

Classification

CML generally progresses through four characteristic stages:

1. Chronic phase. In this phase there are less than 5% blasts and promyelocytes in the peripheral blood or bone marrow. The chronic phase may last for several years without change, but will eventually progress through an accelerated phase to an acute phase.

2. Accelerated phase. In this phase there are less than 30% but greater than 5% blasts in either the peripheral blood or bone marrow. Some 80% of these patients develop a myeloid blast crisis, the management of which is similar to that of AML. The rest develop a lymphoid blast crisis requiring treatment similar to that for ALL.

3. Blast phase. In this phase there are greater then 30% blasts in the peripheral blood or bone marrow. The term blast crisis is used when the patient also has symptoms (fever, malaise, progressive splenomegaly). As described above, this can be either a myeloid or a lymphoid crisis.

4. Meningeal. This is diagnosed by morphological examination of the cerebral spinal fluid (CSF) and the identification of blasts.

Management

Leukapheresis and platelet pheresis may be required to reduce grossly elevated blood counts at presentation.

Chemotherapy

Single-agent chemotherapy with agents such as hydroxyurea and busulphan reduces white-cell number and hence symptoms. Co-administration of allopurinol, to prevent tumour lysis syndrome and gout, is important. Reduction in white-cell number is generally associated with persistence of the Philadelphia chromosome and does not prevent acute transformation.

High-dose chemotherapy and total-body irradiation with allogeneic bone-marrow transplantation may increase overall survival and achieve cure in a small number of cases. All suitable patients should therefore be considered for such treatment while in the chronic phase of their illness when such treatment is most effective.

The results of treatment following blast transformation are poor. Intensive chemotherapy regimes used in acute myeloid or lymphocytic leukaemia rarely achieve prolonged response.

Biological therapy

Interferon-α has been demonstrated to be effective in the management of CML. Complete haematological response (37–84%) and cytogenetic response (15%) has been demonstrated with prolonged therapy. Maintenance interferon-α therapy following reduction of white-cell count with hydroxyurea is therefore increasingly used as first-line therapy for those in whom bone-marrow transplantation is not possible.

Radiotherapy	This may be used to palliate symptoms, for example painful splenomegaly or lytic bone lesions. Total-body irradiation is used in conjunction with high-dose chemotherapy prior to allogeneic transplantation. Cranial irradiation can be used for meningeal disease.
Surgery	Occasionally splenectomy is performed for patients with a massive spleen and with haematological problems.

Prognostic factors

Overall, median survival is approximately 4–5 years. Following blast transformation median survival is a few months. Philadelphia chromosome negativity at presentation is associated with a worse prognosis.

Chronic lymphoid leukaemia

CLL is characterized by the accumulation of large numbers of morphologically mature but immunologically immature lymphocytes.

Incidence	CLL accounts for 25% of all leukaemias. It occurs rarely under the age of 40, with a peak incidence of 60–80 years. The male to female ratio is 2:1.
Aetiology	The aetiology is unknown.
Histology	CLL is characterized by an absolute increase in numbers of lymphocytes in peripheral blood and bone marrow. CLL lymphocytes express characteristic molecules on their cell surface, for example B-cell antigens CD19 and CD20 or the T-cell antigen CD5. CLL may rarely develop into a large cell lymphoma (Richter's syndrome).

Clinical features

Presentation	This may be diagnosed incidentally on routine screening. Common symptoms reflect marrow failure: fatigue, bruising and recurrent infections (hypogammaglobulinaemia). Lymphadenopathy and hepatosplenomegaly may occur.
Investigations	*1. FBC.* Lymphocytosis can present with a white-cell count greater than 300×10^9/l. There may be associated

anaemia (due to bone-marrow suppression, haemolysis or hypersplenism) and thrombocytopaenia.

2. *Serum electrophoresis.* This often shows hypogammaglobulinaemia and may sometimes show a monoclonal band.

Staging   CLL has no standard staging system. The Binet and Rai staging systems are occasionally used.

Management

CLL predominantly affects an elderly population, progresses slowly and is generally considered incurable. Treatment is therefore predominantly given in a conservative fashion.

General   General supportive care is required with prompt antibiotic treatment for infections, steroids for haemolysis and transfusion support when required. Immunogobulin replacement is useful for those who experience repeated infection due to hypogammaglobulinaemia.

Chemotherapy   Symptomatic patients may be treated with single-agent oral chemotherapy. Chlorambucil is effective in reducing tumour bulk in most cases. Cyclophosphamide, fludarabine, deoxycoformycin and chlorodeoxyadenosine are also effective in disease control.

Radiotherapy   Troublesome lymphadenopathy or splenomegaly can be controlled by radiotherapy.

Prognostic factors

Sixty per cent of patients survive 5 years with some living over 10 years, depending on the stage at diagnosis. Younger female patients tend to do better. Death is usually due to bone-marrow failure or infection.

Related topic of interest

Leukaemia – acute (p. 126)

LUNG CANCER

Background

Incidence

This is the commonest cancer in the UK with 40 000 new cases each year, accounting for 1 in 6 of all new cancer cases. Approximately 1 in 11 men will develop lung cancer. Although lung cancer is more common in men, the incidence of lung cancer in women continues to increase.

The incidence is strongly related to age and rises steeply in both men and women after the age of 40.

Risk factors

1. Smoking. Eighty to ninety per cent of cases are caused by smoking and in particular the carcinogenic activity of inhaled tars.

2. Occupation. Asbestos exposure, uranium mining, ship building and petroleum refining.

Aetiology

Chromosomal deletions of 3p and to a lesser extent 13q and 17p. These deletions result in the loss of tumour suppressor genes which probably lead to malignant transformation and tumour progression. The overexpression of many oncogenes such as *ras*, *myc* and *c-erb-b2* is also frequently identified.

Histology

Tumours arise from the epithelium of the large and medium-sized bronchi, rarely from the lung parenchyma itself. The WHO classifies lung tumours as:

- Squamous cell (35-45%).
- Small cell (25%). These are believed to derive from neuro-endocrine cells within the lung. They are therefore often associated with neuro-peptide secretion such as ADH or ACTH.
- Adenocarcinoma (15%). These frequently arise in areas of lung damage, typically peripherally and are more frequent in women.
- Large cell carcinoma (10%).
- Others (5%). These include carcinoid, mesothelioma, sarcoma and lymphoma.

Lung cancer is frequently classified as non-small cell (NSCLC) or small cell (SCLC) due to the distinct clinical features and hence management of SCLC.

It is not clear whether these distinct tumours arise from different cell types or from a single common progenitor which then differentiates to produce different tumour types.

Clinical features

Presentation

The majority of patients present with non-specific symptoms of the primary tumour such as cough, dyspnoea, haemoptysis, chest pain, or recurrent chest infection. As most of these symptoms are common to smokers, late presentation is frequent.

Tumours at specific sites may produce particular syndromes: apical tumours may invade the brachial plexus producing Horner's syndrome and pain in the distribution of the nerve routes involved (Pancoast's syndrome). Recurrent laryngeal nerve palsy and superior vena cava obstruction may be associated with mediastinal disease.

Specific histologies may be associated with a pattern of presentation. Clubbing is more frequent with squamous cell carcinoma. Sputum production may be excessive in bronchiolo-alveolar carcinoma. SCLC may present with manifestations related to the production of neuro-endocrine factors.

A wide variety of paraneoplastic syndromes may occur with lung cancer.

Investigations

CXR. More than 95% of lung tumours are visible on a plain CXR at presentation.

Sputum cytology. Over 80% of patients with lung cancer have malignant cells detectable in the sputum. Identification of the histological sub-type is frequently possible, especially the identification of small-cell tumours.

Bronchoscopy. Fibre-optic or rigid bronchoscopy allows visualization of the bronchial tree, tumour biopsy and bronchial washings to be taken.

Other biopsy techniques. Transthoracic biopsy under radiological guidance is sometimes required for the biopsy of peripheral tumours. Mediastinoscopy and biopsy of abnormal lymph nodes may be important in the assessment of a patient's suitability for surgical resection.

Tumour markers. Neuron-specific enolase (NSE) and lactate dehydrogenase (LDH) may provide useful indications of tumour activity.

To assess accurately the stage of the tumour, CT scans of chest and abdomen and isotopic bone scan are required.

Patients considered for surgical resection require assessment of cardiopulmonary function.

Staging

The TNM staging of lung carcinoma is as follows:

T1	3 cm or less.
T2	More than 3 cm.
T3	Local invasion (operable).
T4	Organ invasion (inoperable).

N1	Bronchopulmonary and hilar nodes.
N2	Ipsilateral mediastinal operable.
N3	Contralateral mediastinal and hilar nodes, supraclavicular nodes inoperable.

M0	No metastases.
M1	Distant metastases.

UICC/AJCC stage grouping for both SCLC and NSCLC is as follows:

Stage 1:	T1, N0, M0.
Stage 2:	T1, N1, M0.
	T2, N1, M0.
Stage 3a:	T3 or N2, M0.
Stage 3b:	T4 or N3, M0.
Stage 4:	M1.

SCLC metastasises extremely early in its clinical course and most patients will have occult metastases at presentation. The TNM classification and stage groupings are therefore not frequently employed in

SCLC. The Veterans Administration Lung Cancer Study Group (VALG) devised a more appropriate staging system as follows:

1. *Limited.* Tumour confined to one hemi-thorax with local extension confined to ipsilateral or contralateral mediastinal or supraclavicular lymph nodes.

2. *Extensive.* Disease at sites beyond the definition of limited disease. Two thirds of patients present with extensive disease.

Management

The management of SCLC and NSCLC is different and will therefore be considered separately.

Small cell lung cancer

Surgery

The early dissemination of SCLC means it should be considered a systemic disease at presentation. Surgical intervention is therefore inappropriate for 90% of cases. Patients with tumours less than 3 cm in diameter with nodal disease confined to bronchopulmonary and hilar nodes may be considered for surgical resection

Radiotherapy

SCLC is a radiosensitive tumour. There are three indications for radiotherapy in the management of SCLC:

1. *Treatment of primary tumour.* A recent meta-analysis of thoracic radiotherapy in addition to chemotherapy demonstrated a 5% survival advantage at 3 years in patients with limited disease. Local control is achieved with radiation such that relapse occurs at a site distant to that of the primary disease.

2. *Prophylactic cranial irradiation (PCI).* Brain metastases are frequent in SCLC and cause significant morbidity. PCI reduces the frequency of brain metastases but has not been associated with a significant increase in overall survival. PCI is associated with toxicities such as

memory impairment, functional deficit and dementia and it is therefore not routinely administered to all patients.

3. Palliative. Radiotherapy may be used to palliate the symptoms of advanced SCLC which is unresponsive to other treatments.

Chemotherapy

SCLC is one of the most chemosensitive solid tumours. Chemotherapy is therefore the mainstay of SCLC management with responses occurring within days. Complications such as superior vena cava obstruction (SVCO) or spinal cord compression can be treated with chemotherapy rather than radiotherapy. This is in contrast to NSCLC.

Ninety per cent of patients with SCLC will respond to combination chemotherapy with complete response rates approaching 50%. Standard regimes include:

- Vincristine/doxorubicin/cyclophosphamide.
- Ifosfamide/carboplatin/etoposide.
- Methotrexate/vinblastine/carboplatin.
- Cisplatin/etoposide.
- Etoposide.

Most patients who relapse will do so within 12 months of chemotherapy, with disease that is chemo-resistant, and die from rapidly progressive disease.

Prognostic factors

Without treatment, SCLC has an extremely bad prognosis, with a median survival of 2–4 months. For patients treated with systemic chemotherapy, the median survival is approximately 11 months (limited disease, 10–16 months; extensive disease, 6–12 months).

Prognostic factors include extent of disease at presentation, number of metastatic sites, performance status, degree of weight loss and biochemical abnormalities (elevated LDH or low sodium or albumin).

Patients with limited disease, a good performance status, and favourable biochemistry have a small but real chance of long-term survival (10–15%). Patients with extensive disease who are less fit are rarely cured but can obtain good palliation from chemotherapy.

Non-small cell lung cancer

Most patients with NSCLC are dead within 12 months of diagnosis. However, the prognosis is better in selected groups and active anti-cancer treatment may be appropriate.

Surgery

Stage 1 and 2 (T1–2, N0–1) NSCLC managed with surgical resection has a good prognosis (80% 5 year survival with T1, N0 disease) and the possibility of cure. Mediastinal involvement is considered a contraindication to surgery by most surgeons. Approximately 30% of NSCLC are suitable for surgery.

There is a 3–5% mortality with a pneumonectomy. More limited resections such as lobectomy or wedge resections are therefore performed if possible.

Following surgery, adjuvant radiotherapy or chemotherapy may be indicated.

Radiotherapy

In patients not suitable for surgery, radical radiotherapy produces 20% 5 year survival for patients with stage 1 or 2 disease. Randomized controlled trials comparing continuous, hyperfractionated accelerated radiotherapy (CHART) with conventional radiotherapy are ongoing in the UK.

Adjuvant chemotherapy following radical radiotherapy is associated with minimal improvements in survival.

Palliative radiotherapy is used frequently and is the first-line treatment for complications of brain metastases, superior vena cava obstruction or spinal cord compression.

Chemotherapy

Chemotherapy can produce response rates of up to 45% (11% complete response rate) with combination regimes such as mitomycin C, ifosfamide and cisplatin. However, a recent meta-analysis demonstrated response duration to be short and the survival advantage limited. Chemotherapy has therefore not been offered routinely to patients. Current randomized trials address this issue.

Chemotherapy may be given as an adjuvant to surgery or radical radiotherapy. The meta-analysis demonstrated limited benefits.

Neoadjuvant chemotherapy prior to surgery has been demonstrated in a randomized trial to improve overall survival in some patients.

Prognostic factors

Stage of tumour

Stage 1:	50%	5 year survival.
Stage 2:	40%	5 year survival.
Stage 3a:	25%	5 year survival.
Stage 3b:	<5%	5 year survival.
Stage 4:		median survival is less than 6 months.

Current issues

Chemotherapy

The role of chemotherapy for the management of NSCLC is being addressed by a large multicentre trial, 'The Big Lung Trial', which aims to recruit 9000 patients.

Further reading

Non-small cell lung cancer collaborative group. Chemotherapy in non-small cell lung cancer: a meta analysis using updated data on individual patients from 52 randomised clinical trials. *British Medical Journal*, 1995; **311:** 899–909.

Related topics of interest

Paraneoplastic syndromes (p. 201)
Smoking (p. 241)

MELANOMA – MALIGNANT

Malignant melanoma is a malignant tumour arising from melanocytes.

Background

Incidence

In the UK, malignant melanoma accounts for 4% of malignancies, with an annual incidence of approximately 50 per million and almost 3000 new cases per year. It is more common in females (2:1 female:male ratio). Melanoma is relatively more common in young adults than most other cancers, accounting for 22% of malignancies occurring before the age of 40 years. The incidence in the UK and worldwide has been steadily rising over the last 25 years with a doubling in incidence in the last 10 years.

Aetiology

Sunlight is the main aetiological agent. Exposure to sunlight is more significant in childhood, especially high intensity, intermittent exposure which causes sunburn. This is consistent with the increased incidence of melanoma in fair-skinned populations (melanin pigment is protective) and in hot countries (e.g. Australia) where the incidence is as high as 500 per million in certain areas.

Familial predisposition may account for up to 5% of melanomas. The majority of familial melanoma cases are part of an autosomal dominant dysplastic naevus syndrome characterized by multiple dysplastic naevii and a increased risk of malignant melanoma (× 400). An inherited loss of the *p16* tumour-suppressor gene has been identified recently in some families.

Histology

Five main clinical lesions are seen:

- Superficial spreading 70%.
- Nodular 15–30%.
- Lentigo maligna 5–10%.
- Acral lentigious 2%.
- Ocular melanoma less than 1%.

These are predominantly descriptive terms. However, the management and prognosis are dependent more on the thickness of the lesion than on the above subtype.

The sequence of progression of melanoma is thought to be an initial phase of horizontal growth, followed by vertical growth invading through the dermis. There is then spread through the lymphatics and the bloodstream to distant sites.

Clinical features

Presentation

The majority of patients present with a change in character of a pre-existing pigmented lesion. Changes in the size, shape or colour of an existing lesion or three of the following should be considered with suspicion:

- Diameter greater than 7 mm.
- Inflammation.
- Oozing/crusting.
- Itching.
- Bleeding.

A minority of patients will present with symptoms relating to their metastases. Melanoma can metastasize to any site in the body. More common sites include lymph nodes, subcutaneous tissue, lung, liver, bone or brain.

Investigations

Excision biopsy. Confirms the diagnosis and gives the depth of invasion.

Radiological staging. CXR and abdominal ultrasound or CT scanning of the chest, abdomen and pelvis assesses the degree of distant spread.

Staging

Two pathological staging systems are generally used:

- Breslow's (measures vertical thickness of lesion in mm).
- Clarke's (describes anatomic level of invasion):

Stage I: epidermis only.
Stage II: papillary dermis.
Stage III: fills and expands papillary dermis.
Stage IV: invasion into reticular dermis.
Stage V: invasion into subcutaneous tissue.

There are several clinical staging systems for melanoma, but the most widely used is the AJCC staging:

Stage I: localized lesion, less than 1.5 mm thick.
Stage II: localized lesion greater than 1.5 mm thick.
Stage III: regional lymph nodes.
Stage IV: distant metastases.

Management

Surgery

This is the mainstay of curative therapy. A wide local excision of the primary lesion should be performed either as the primary procedure or following the excision biopsy. The minimum margins of excision depend on the thickness of the tumour. A 1 cm margin has been shown to be sufficient for lesions less than 2 mm thick. This usually allows primary closure and obviates the need for a split skin graft. For thicker lesions, 3 cm margins are generally considered sufficient but the matter is presently the subject of clinical trials.

Some patients with regional lymph nodes at presentation or relapse can be cured with radical lymph node resection. However, elective lymph node dissection for stage I and II disease of the limbs is not indicated, as demonstrated in several large studies.

Radiotherapy

Melanoma is a relatively radioresistant malignancy, and the main role for radiotherapy is in the palliation of symptomatic brain, bone and soft tissue metastases.

Chemotherapy

Melanoma is generally a drug-resistant cancer. Dacarbazine (DTIC), cisplatin, the nitrosureas (BCNU and CCNU) and vinblastine are the most active agents, with single agent response rates of only 15–20%. These responses last for 5–6 months, but give only limited survival benefit.

Combinations of these therapies have been used in regimens such as BOLD (BCNU/vincristine/lomustine DTIC) and CVD (cisplatin/vinblastine/DTIC). These can increase the response rate to 30–40% but again with little survival benefit. The addition of tamoxifen to chemotherapy appears to have a therapeutic effect.

Biological therapies IFN-α has a response rate of approximately 15% when used alone. Its use in an adjuvant setting is being tested for high-risk patients. IL-2 has been studied extensively in melanoma with response rates of up to 20% being reported. Some of these have been durable responses lasting several years.

A range of vaccine strategies have been tried with little benefit so far.

Screening

There is no screening of the general population but screening of at-risk individuals is being assessed. There is a public awareness campaign to discourage excessive sun exposure.

Current issues

Tumour antigens have been identified in melanoma that can be recognized by patient's cytotoxic T cells. This has led to several new approaches to enhance the immune response which include gene therapy and peptide vaccines.

Further reading

Schuchter M. Melanoma and other skin neoplasms, *Current Opinion in Oncology*, 1997; 175–77.

Related topics of interest

Biological therapy (p. 7)
Immunotherapy (p. 119)
Interleukin-2 (p. 123)

METASTASES

The dissemination of a malignant tumour may occur by local invasion or metastasis. Metastatic spread classically occurs by lymphatic, haematogenous or trans-coelomic spread across body cavities.

Biology of metastasis

The ability of solid tumours to metastasize requires:

- Breach of basement membrane.
- Stromal invasion.
- Invasion into vascular or lymphatic structures.
- Dissemination to distant sites.
- Extravasation from vascular or lymphatic structures.
- Growth in the foreign tissue environment.

The activation of oncogenes or inactivation of tumour suppressor genes both of which confer a growth advantage on cells, are generally insufficient to achieve these processes. Additional discrete genetic changes and subsequent phenotypic change are required.

Important examples include:

- Adhesion molecules: leading to loss of cell–cell interactions.
- Angiogenic factors: secretion leads to new vessel formation.
- Metalloproteinases: secretion leads to dissolving of the extra-cellular matrix.

Clinical aspects of metastasis

Site

The most frequent sites of metastatic disease are:

Pulmonary. These tumours come most commonly from lung, breast and kidney.

Hepatic. These tumours come most commonly from colorectal, breast and lung.

Bone. These tumours are generally from lung, breast, prostate, kidney and infrequently from thyroid.

Other sites of metastatic disease are frequently associated with particular primary tumours, for example

	adrenal metastases from a small-cell lung cancer primary.
Treatment	The identification of metastatic disease has profound implications for the management of patients with cancer. In the majority of solid tumours, metastatic disease implies incurable disease. Palliative treatment is therefore given systemically (chemotherapy) or locally (radiotherapy or surgery).
	In certain clinical situations metastatic disease may still be treated aggressively with curative intent. Germ-cell tumours are highly chemosensitive and intensive combination chemotherapy may still achieve cure despite widely metastatic disease. Surgical intervention with curative intent is more controversial. Resection of liver metastases in patients with colorectal carcinoma and lung metastases in patients with soft-tissue sarcoma may achieve cure for a number of patients.

Prognostic factors

The presence of metastatic disease is an adverse prognostic factor for all malignancies. The extent of dissemination also correlates with prognosis; metastasis to regional lymph nodes is associated with a better prognosis than distant spread.

Current issues

Early diagnosis	The detection of sub-clinical metastatic disease has implications for the management of malignancy. The detection of circulating tumours cells with the polymerase chain reaction or immunohistochemical means is being investigated.
Treatment	New anti-cancer therapies aimed at inhibiting the metastatic process including metalloproteinase inhibitors and anti-angiogenesis agents are being developed.

METHOTREXATE

Methotrexate is an anti-metabolite cytotoxic drug. Effective anti-metabolites such as methotrexate and 5-FU interfere with key enzymes involved principally in the synthesis of DNA and RNA.

Uses

Methotrexate is frequently used in combination with other chemotherapeutic agents in the management of a diverse range of primary malignancies such as leukaemia, lymphoma, breast and bladder carcinoma, and sarcoma. Methotrexate is safely administered intrathecally and therefore can be used to treat disease within the meninges.

Methotrexate is used as a maintenance therapy in the management of acute childhood leukaemias.

The immunosuppresive properties of methotrexate are exploited in the management of autoimmune diseases such as rheumatoid arthritis.

Mode of action

Methotrexate is a derivative of folinic acid. It competitively inhibits the cytoplasmic enzyme dihydrofolate reductase, leading to an inhibition of nucleotide synthesis. Specificity to tumour cells reflects their increased rate of proliferation. Immunosuppression results from inhibition of lymphocyte proliferation.

Pharmacokinetics

Methotrexate is renally excreted, with the majority cleared within 6 hours of intravenous administration. Methotrexate diffuses into 'third-space' fluid collections such as ascites and pleural effusions. Subsequent reabsorption of the drug from these spaces into the circulation may lead to a prolonged effect and hence increased toxicity. Therefore such effusions should be drained prior to methotrexate administration.

Methotrexate serum levels and hence toxicity are altered by concomitant medication with drugs which affect its protein binding within the serum or renal excretion (e.g. NSAIDs).

Scheduling

Methotrexate is given orally, intravenously or intrathecally. Doses are calculated relative to the patient's surface area.

With higher doses or where previous toxicity has occured, folinic acid can be administered to reduce side effects. This 'folinic acid rescue' is generally given as oral medication, beginning 24 hours after methotrexate administration, for 24–72 hours.

In patients receiving high-dose methotrexate, adequate hydration and urinary alkalinization are important to ensure renal excretion of the drug. Folinic acid rescue is continued until serum methotrexate levels fall to safe levels.

Toxicity

1. Myelosuppression. Myelosuppression occurs frequently, resulting in thrombocytopenia, anaemia or leukopenia. It represents the dose-limiting toxicity and therefore, with appropriate haematological support, dose escalation is possible.

2. Nausea and vomiting. This is frequently controlled with the use of standard anti-emetics such as metoclopramide.

3. Alopecia. This occurs infrequently.

4. Gastrointestinal toxicity. Mucositis is a common toxicity. It can be severe, occasionally leading to intestinal haemorrhage and perforation.

5. Hepatic toxicity. Prolonged administration or high-dose therapy can cause hepatic damage.

6. Central nervous system. A variety of CNS toxicities have been reported ranging from headache, alteration of mood and drowsiness to a leukoencephalopathy.

MOLECULAR BIOLOGY OF CANCER

Cancer results from an accumulation of multiple genetic alterations that either inhibit or enhance normal cellular processes. Through a process of continual genetic 'evolution' a cell acquires new phenotypes able to proliferate, invade, disseminate throughout the body, escape immune surveillance and resist treatment.

Many genetic alterations have been recognized in human tumours. Some of these confer a survival advantage and hence lead to clonal expansion of the founder cell. Most are frequent events (e.g. *p53* mutation) found in a wide variety of tumours. Other genetic aberrations are clearly related to individual tumours and either reflect the predisposition in such tissues to these genetic changes or the alterations required to overcome that tissue's normal regulatory control.

Cancer genes

Many genes whose alteration is associated with carcinogenesis have been identified. Although initally known as oncogenes, the identification of inhibitory genes has led to the classification of cancer genes as either oncogenes or tumour suppressor genes.

Oncogenes

Oncogenes are derived from normal physiological genes (proto-oncogenes) which control normal cell function. More than 100 oncogenes have been identified. Many proto-oncogenes form components of signal transduction pathways which transmit growth signals from the cell membrane to the nucleus. Oncogenes have been identified in human tumours which affect most components of signal transduction pathways such as growth factor receptors (*ERB-B2*), GTP-binding proteins (ras) and nuclear transcription factors (myc). Proto-oncogenes become activated by:

1. Mutation. Alterations of the nucleotide sequence lead to either an alteration in the amino acid sequence, or premature termination of translation may produce a protein with abnormal function.

2. Chromosomal rearrangement. Chromosomal translocations may lead to the formation of a novel fusion protein or loss of normal control of proto-oncogene expression.

3. Amplification. Multiple copies of a proto-oncogene, may result from dysregulated chromosomal replication. This in turn may lead to inappropriate high levels of expression.

Examples of oncogenes frequently affected in human cancer are:

- *ras:* the ras pathway is central to the transmission of a growth factor signal from cell membrane to nucleus. Activation of the three *ras* genes (*Ha-ras, Ki-ras, N-ras*) by point mutation is the most frequent dominant oncogene abnormality in human cancer. *ras* mutations are frequently seen in bladder, lung and colorectal carcinoma.
- *myc:* the *myc* family of genes (*c-myc, L-myc, N-myc*) are frequently activated by amplification to form oncogenes. Myc in combination with associated proteins (MAX, MAD) acts as a transcription factor controlling the expression of genes associated with cell division. *myc* amplification is associated with many tumours such as small-cell lung carcinoma and neuroblastoma. A chromosomal translocation in Burkitt's lymphoma leads to *c-myc* activation.
- *Mdm-2:* mdm-2 has recently been identified as an oncogene which does not produce a component of the transduction pathway of a growth signal. The mdm-2 protein acts by binding and inactivating genes such as *p53* (an example of an oncogene affecting a tumour suppressor gene). *Mdm-2* overexpression has been identified in soft tissue sarcomas.

Tumour suppressor genes These are defined as genes in which mutation or other genetic modification leads to a loss of function which is then associated with tumour formation. The normal function of the protein product of these genes is generally central to the control of cell division and differentiation. Typically, both copies of a tumour suppressor gene must be affected to lead to loss of the protein's function, that is, the gene acts recessively.

Inactivation of a tumour suppressor gene may result from:

1. Deletion. Deletion of both copies of a tumour suppressor gene (homozygous deletion) may occur. Deletion of a single copy with inactivation of the other allele by alternative means is the most frequent mechanism leading to inactivation of a tumour suppressor gene. The detection of the single remaining allele by molecular techniques leads to a loss of heterozygosity, the characteristic marker of a region of the genome in which tumour suppressor gene is located.

2. Mutation. Mutation of one or both alleles may result in tumour suppressor gene inactivation.

3. Epigenetic. Inactivation of a tumour suppressor gene by means which do not alter the genetic sequence of the genome are known as epigenetic changes. For example, inappropriate methylation may lead to a loss of expression and hence inactivation of the cell cycle regulator *p16*.

A small number of genes has been identified which act as tumour suppressor genes. These include:

- *p53:* the protein product of the *p53* gene has a molecular weight of 53 kDa and is central to the control of the cell cycle and the response of the cell to stress such as DNA damage. *p53* functions principally by controlling transcription of other genes which control pathways such as the cell cycle, DNA repair and apoptosis. Loss of normal *p53* function is central to the pathogenesis of many malignancies; *p53* mutations are the most common identified in human cancer, present in more than 50% of tumours. Germ-line deletion of one copy of the *p53* gene leads to an increase in tumour incidence (Li–Fraumeni syndrome).
- *pRb:* the retinoblastoma gene (*Rb1*) produces a protein with an essential role in the control of the cell cycle; loss of normal function leads to a loss of control of the G1/S checkpoint and hence inappropriate proliferation.

Carcinogenesis

A single genetic defect is rarely sufficient to produce an overt malignancy. The majority of tumours follow the accumulation of multiple genetic abnormalities. This multi-step genetic model of tumourigenesis is best characterized for colorectal carcinoma. More than seven genetic defects have been identified which are associated with the progression from normal epithelium to carcinoma and include the oncogene, *K-ras* and tumour suppressor genes *APC, p53* and *DCC*.

Clinical implications

Prognosis

The identification of specific genetic defects may have prognostic significance; abnormal *p53* protein in bladder cancer is associated with a poorer prognosis.

Treatment

It is hoped that a clearer understanding of the molecular biology of cancer will lead to improvements in cancer therapy. The correction of the underlying genetic defects may reverse the malignant phenotype and lead to resolution of the tumour, for example the injection of wild-type *p53* into lung tumours.

Current issues

Gene discovery

The identification of new cancer genes, in particular those that initiate the earliest malignant change, is a subject under intense investigation.

Treatment

The identification of the specific defects in cells which underly the malignant, invasive or metastatic phenotype is enabling the development of novel anti-cancer therapies.

Further reading

Yarnold JR, Stratton MR, Macmillan TJ, *Molecular Biology for Oncology,* 2nd edn. Chapman and Hall, 1996.

Related topics of interest

Apoptosis (p. 4)
Gene therapy (p. 102)

MORPHINE

Morphine is the main naturally occurring alkaloid of opium. Diamorphine is a semi-synthetic analogue of morphine which is rapidly converted to morphine following administration.

Uses

Morphine is the drug of choice for continuous cancer pain (i.e. visceral and soft tissue pain). It is much less effective for other pains such as bone and nerve (neuropathic) pain, although it can have a role (morphine partially responsive pain). Colicky pain does not respond to morphine (morphine non-responsive pain). The appropriate use of co-analgesics and other interventions will be necessary in morphine partially responsive pain and non-responsive pain.

Morphine can also be used to palliate dyspnoea in cancer patients either systemically or, more contentiously, via a nebulizer.

Morphine is not used as a sedative or hypnotic. Other drugs such as benzodiazepines and neuroleptics are clinically indicated in this situation.

Mode of action

Morphine acts on opioid receptors which have been demonstrated both within and outside the CNS. The receptors outside the CNS are located in the iris, the bronchial epithelium and the gut. CNS receptors are present in both the brain and spinal cord. The major receptor subtypes are μ, δ and κ. Analgesia is mediated via μ and δ receptors within the CNS. The function of κ receptor is less clear.

Pharmacokinetics

1. Bioavailability. Morphine is completely absorbed from the GI tract, predominantly in the proximal small bowel. There is extensive pre-systemic elimination which accounts for the reduced bioavailability of morphine after oral administration.

2. Metabolism. The primary site of morphine metabolism is the liver. The main metabolites are morphine-3-glucuronide (M3G) and morphine-6-glucuronide (M6G). Significantly decreased liver function is required to increase the bioavailability of morphine and have a clinical impact. M6G is believed to account for much of the analgesic activity of morphine.

3. Excretion. The main route of excretion for morphine (and its metabolites) is through the kidney by glomerular filtration. Renal impairment will lead to morphine accumulation and a reduction of dosage and frequency of administration may be necessary. The plasma elimination half-life of morphine is 2–4 hours.

Scheduling

1. Oral. This is the optimal and preferred route of administration. Available preparations of oral morphine include:

- Immediate-release morphine solution.
- Immediate-release morphine tablets.
- Slow-release 12 hourly morphine tablets and suspension.
- Slow-release once daily morphine tablets.

The basic rules of administration are:
(a) Start with an immediate release morphine preparation for ease of dose titration.
(b) Give every 4 hours (continued through the night or give a double dose at night).
(c) Starting doses: 5–10 mg every 4 hours if the patient has previously been taking weak opiods; 2.5 mg every four hours for elderly or opioid naïve patients.
(d) Review regularly and increase the dose until pain free for the full 4 hours.
(e) Dose increments of 30–50% dependent on both the response and side effects.
(f) If pain free and drowsy, dose reduction may be necessary.
(g) Once a stable dose of immediate release morphine is achieved, convert to maintenance treatment with controlled release morphine for ease of administration and compliance.
(h) For breakthrough pain it is recommended to give 50–100% of the 4-hourly dose as immediate release morphine.
(i) Start a laxative from day 1 (e.g. codanthrusate or codanthramer).

2. *Parenteral.* This route should only be used when oral administration is unreliable or not possible. Diamorphine is the drug of choice because of its high solubility. Methods of administration include:

- Subcutaneous infusion (via a syringe driver).
- Subcutaneous bolus injections (intramuscular injections are painful and unnecessary).
- Intravenous infusion.
- Epidural and intrathecal infusion.
- Transdermal (Fentanyl).

Subcutaneous infusions achieve a steady plasma concentration of the drug without the need for regular injections. They are particularly useful in patients with vomiting, dysphagia, intestinal obstruction, malabsorption or a decreased level of consciousness and are therefore frequently used in the care of dying patients. Intravenous administration is preferred in patients with generalized oedema, a coagulation disorder or poor peripheral circulation.

Dose conversion

Oral morphine and oral diamorphine are of similar potency.

For repeated doses or continuous parenteral infusions (subcutaneous or intravenous) the relative potency of oral morphine to parenteral diamorphine is in the range 1:2–1:3 (e.g. a total of 60 mg oral morphine over 24 hours is equivalent to 20–30 mg of diamorphine in 24 hours as a parenteral infusion). The ratio is higher with bolus intravenous doses of diamorphine because of the greater peak effects.

Side effects

1. *Respiratory depression.* Potentially the most serious adverse effect of strong opioids. If morphine is given chronically and titrated to relieve pain, respiratory depression occurs to a minimal extent, if at all. In using morphine to control dyspnoea there is evidence that it reduces the sensation of dyspnoea proportionally more than it reduces ventilation.

2. *Nausea and vomiting.* All opioids can produce nausea and vomiting by stimulation of the chemoreceptor trigger zone. More than one third of patients will experience nausea and vomiting although

in many it is an initiation side effect and will resolve with continued use. If nausea persists, haloperidol may be effective. Morphine can also delay gastric emptying and occasionally a pro-kinetic drug is indicated to relieve nausea and vomiting. If nausea becomes a persistent problem, switching to an alternative opioid may be necessary.

3. Constipation. Morphine and other opioids decrease colonic activity and cause subsequent constipation. All patients receiving opioids require a laxative to prevent constipation. Codanthramer and codanthrusate are appropriate laxatives. Metoclopramide and cisapride may be useful in opioid-induced constipation.

4. Dry mouth. Opioids reduce GI secretions and may be the cause of a dry mouth. However, other causes must be considered (anti-cholinergics, dehydration, oral infections). It can be managed by regular mouth care and artificial saliva.

5. Neuropsychological effects. Opioid analgesics produce sedation and drowsiness, frequently seen at the start of treatment, which commonly resolve within the first few days. An explanation of this to patients will promote compliance. In patients on stable doses of morphine there is normal cognitive function. Transient drowsiness and cognitive impairment may occur with dose increases. Morphine does not cause euphoria. Any improvement in mood is probably secondary to pain relief.

6. Addiction. In the presence of chronic cancer pain addiction to morphine is very unlikely. In this group of patients the reason for an increase in the dose of morphine is usually an increase in the pain due to tumour growth. This is not tolerance to morphine.

7. Myoclonus. Myoclonic jerks are usually an indication that the dose is inappropriately high or has been increased too rapidly. They may disappear on dose stabilization.

Opioid toxicity   Indicators of opioid toxicity include, visual hallucinations, decreased level of consciousness, respiratory depression and myoclonic jerks. Myosis is a common in 'non-toxic' patients and is not a reliable indicator of toxicity. Severe toxicity may be cautiously reversed by naloxone infusions. Renal failure can cause opioid toxicity even when the dose has been stable for some time as opioid metabolites (notably M6G) are renally excreted.

Current issues

For a small number of patients for whom standard analgesic regimes are poorly tolerated and/or ineffective, newer opioids (hydromorphone, fentanyl patches) should be considered.

Further reading

Expert Working Group of the European Association for Palliative Care. Morphine in cancer pain: modes of administration. *British Medical Journal*, 1996; **312:** 823–6.

Related topic of interest

Pain control in cancer (p. 191)

MULTIPLE MYELOMA

Plasma cell neoplasms may result in a spectrum of diseases ranging from a benign monoclonal gammopathy (BMG) to plasmacytoma and multiple myeloma. Both BMG and plasmacytoma may undergo transformation to malignant myeloma.

Background

Incidence   Approximately 3000 cases of multiple myleoma occur in the UK each year, representing 1% of all cancers. The peak incidence occurs at 75 years with 90% occurring after the age of 50. The disease is commoner in males (1.4:1).

Risk factors   There is an association with farming and chemical or radiation exposure.

Aetiology   The cause of multiple myeloma is unknown. However, frequent abnormalities of various chromosomes (commonly 8) and oncogenes (*c-myc*) are recognized.

Histology   Multiple myeloma arises from a neoplastic transformation of plasma cells. These malignant cells are large, have immature nuclei, and may proliferate in the bone marrow, in a localized mass (plasmacytoma) or in peripheral blood.

Myeloma cells are characterized by secretion of immunoglobulin (Ig) chains (paraprotein). Sixty per cent of patients have an IgG paraprotein, 20% IgA. Other Ig classes are rare.

In 25% the light chain only is produced (kappa or lambda). This protein is filtered by the glomerulus, and can be detected in urine when it is known as the 'Bence–Jones' protein.

Clinical features

Diagnosis of multiple myeloma requires at least two of the following characteristics:

* Monoclonal immunoglobulin in the blood or urine.
* Malignant plasma cells within the bone marrow (>10%).
* Osteolytic bone lesions.

Presentation

Frequently presenting features include bone pain (70%), hypercalcaemia (20%), anaemia (15%), infections (15%) and renal impairment (20%).

Investigations

To confirm diagnosis:

- Protein electrophoresis of the blood and urine; to detect and analyse a paraprotein.
- Bone-marrow aspiration and trephine biopsy.
- Skeletal survey of plain X-rays to detect the characteristic punched-out lesions of myeloma. These may occur anywhere, particularly in the long bones, skull vault and mandible.

To detect complications:

- Full blood count and plasma viscosity.
- Urea and electrolytes.
- Glomerular filtration rate.
- Serum corrected calcium.
- Serum alkaline phosphatase, which is typically normal in the absence of fractures.

Staging

Multiple myeloma is staged according to the Medical Research Council (MRC) scale on the basis of three factors:

- Stage I: all of the following: blood urea < 8.0 mM, Hb > 10 g/dl, performance status 0 or 1.
- Stage II: not stage I or II.
- Stage III: two of the following: blood urea > 10.0 mM, Hb < 7.5 g/dl, performance status 3 or 4.

Management

Patients with 'smouldering myeloma' often have few clinical problems and stable disease. They do not benefit from treatment at this stage.

General measures

Good symptom control is important. In particular, adequate hydration with at least 3 l of fluid is required daily to avoid symptoms associated with hypercalcaemia, hyperviscosity and renal impairment.

Radiotherapy

Radiotherapy is the treatment of choice for painful bony lesions.

Chemotherapy	Chemotherapy is indicated in symptomatic or progressive disease.

In patients with a poor performance status, a combination of melphalan and prednisolone is associated with a 50% response with minimal toxicity. Median survival is improved from 7 to 21 months.

In fitter patients response rates of 60% can be achieved with combinations containing BCNU and doxorubicin. Median survival is increased to 28 months, but toxicity is greater.

Second-line treatment with infusional chemotherapy (vincristine, doxorubicin, and methylprednisolone) has a role following relapse. |
| **Biological therapy** | Low-dose interferon-α has been demonstrated to prolong remissions and increase survival following chemotherapy. |

Prognostic factors

Cure is uncommon. Median survival is 2–3 years, with few patients surviving beyond 10 years.

The following correlate to prognosis in multivariate analysis:

- Serum β_2-microglobulin. This is the most significant prognostic indicator.
- Performance status.
- Haemoglobin.
- Renal function.

Current issues

High-dose chemotherapy	The role of intensive chemotherapy with bone-marrow support is the focus of a MRC trial.

Further reading

Drug therapy: the treatment of multiple myeloma. *New England Journal of Medicine*, 1994; **330**: 484–89.

Related topic of interest

Hypercalcaemia (p. 116)

MYELOSUPPRESSION

Myelosuppression is commonly seen in cancer, either as a consequence of disease or, more commonly, as a consequence of treatment. Significant morbidity can result from the complications of this.

Aetiology

Treatment related

Many of the cytotoxic agents that are used to treat malignancy are toxic to the bone marrow and hence cause deficiencies of peripheral blood cells. Most myelosuppressive chemotherapy at conventional doses results in a transient fall in the leukocyte and platelet count. The lowest point, the nadir, generally occurs at about 10–12 days (but may occur at up to 3 weeks with some drugs). Recovery generally occurs over a similar period due to maturation of blood cell precursors. With higher doses of chemotherapy the fall in total leukocyte count is more profound and more sustained. Different agents have differential effects on different components of the bone marrow; for example carboplatin causes relatively more thrombocytopenia. Myelosupression is also seen with biological therapies such as interferon and interleukin-2, but the mechanisms and kinetics differ from that caused by conventional chemotherapy.

Bone marrow infiltration

Bone marrow replacement by malignant infiltration can produce pancytopenia. This is more with common haematological malignancies and certain solid cancers, for example breast cancer and lung cancer. Successful anti-tumour therapy will lead to an improvement in the pancytopenia. The use of myelosuppressive cytotoxic agents requires careful consideration and management.

Paraneoplastic syndrome

Pancytopenia is occasionally seen but can also affect individual haematopoietic lineages.

Other

Blood loss from a tumour can also be a cause of anaemia. Other general medical causes also apply to these patients and should be included in the differential diagnosis.

Investigation

A transient nadir in blood counts following chemotherapy can be observed. However, prolonged or excessive degrees of suppression require investigation to exclude alternative causes such as marrow infiltration. Full evaluation includes a blood film, measurement of haematinics, bone-marrow aspirate and trephine.

Treatment

Anaemia

A haemoglobin level less than 10 g/dl, especially in the presence of symptoms, may require blood transfusion. The use of erythropoietin in preventing symptomatic anaemia is being investigated.

Thrombocytopenia

Platelet counts less than $10 \times 10^9/l$ are associated with a significant risk of spontaneous bleeding such as intra-cerebral haemorrhage. In the presence of other complications such as infection, platelet counts $10-20 \times 10^9/l$ are frequently supported with platelet transfusion. Platelet counts greater than $20 \times 10^9/l$, in the absence of spontaneous bleeding, rarely require platelet transfusion. Clinical signs of significant thrombocytopenia include petechial haemorrhage, spontaneous nose bleeds, corneal haemorrhage and haematuria. Conventional doses of chemotherapy rarely cause clinically important thrombocytopenia. The use of high-dose chemotherapy is associated with prolonged thrombocytopenia requiring regular platelet transfusions. Repeated administration of blood products such as platelets is associated with the development of specific antibodies to blood cells including platelets. This manifests as a failure to increase platelet counts immediately after transfusion. This suggests the need for single donor (rather than pooled) or HLA matched platelets.

Neutropenia

The most frequent cause of morbidity and mortality associated with myelosuppression is due to neutropenic sepsis. A patient who becomes pyrexial following cytotoxic chemotherapy requires immediate review to assess the degree of neutropenia. Total white counts less than $1 \times 10^9/l$ with an associated fever require immediate in-patient management with broad spectrum antibiotics. Neutropenic patients may not have a raised temperature despite overwhelming sepsis but present feeling non-specifically unwell.

Extensive cultures of blood, urine, sputum, throat and a chest X-ray are taken, and may influence subsequent changes to antibiotic therapy. Although the identification of a causative organism allows modification of antibiotics, broad-spectrum cover is required. A failure to culture organisms is frequent, but 5 days of broad-spectrum antibiotics are usually required. Failure to respond to initial antibiotics within approximately 48 hours requires a change to second-line broad-spectrum antibiotics. Persistent fever despite appropriate antibiotic treatment requires consideration of additional antifungal or antiviral agents.

Failure to instigate prompt and appropriate antibiotic therapy may quickly lead to multi-organ failure associated with septic shock. Patients receiving myelosuppressive chemotherapy must be warned about these potential hazards and the need to seek immediate medical attention in the event of fever. Asymptomatic neutropenia may be closely observed without the need for antibiotics.

Prolonged neutropenia seen with high-dose chemotherapy requires special consideration. Gut sterilization may be used and prophylactic anti-viral agents commenced prior to the neutropenia developing. Atypical infections such as pneumocystis pneumonia (PCP) and systemic fungal or viral infections may occur.

Prevention

Prophylactic antibiotics

The use of prophylactic antibiotics to prevent neutropenic sepsis is not generally required, but in certain conditions should be considered, for example in the presence of chronic obstructive airways disease and the use of cotrimazole in patients with lymphoma at risk of PCP.

Dose modifications

Severe myelosuppression, particularly in association with sepsis, may require subsequent dose reduction of chemotherapy. In patients receiving potentially curative chemotherapy, such as for Hodgkin's disease and testicular cancer, every effort is made to maintain dose intensity. For patients receiving palliative chemotherapy the balance may favour dose reduction.

Colony-stimulating factors The routine use of elective colony-stimulating factors to prevent or reduce neutropenia is not proven to be of benefit. In some patients such use is appropriate as if enables dose intensity to be maintained.

Current issues

The role of colony-stimulating growth factors and erythropoietin continues to be investigated in the prevention of myelosuppression. Thrombopoietin (a platelet growth factor) has recently been described and is being assessed in early clinical studies.

Related topics of interest

Chemotherapy – (a) general principles (p. 48)
Chemotherapy – (b) combination (p. 52)
Chemotherapy – (d) complications (p. 58)

NAUSEA AND VOMITING

Nausea and vomiting (emesis) are frequently associated with both cancer and its treatment. Vomiting occurs in approximately 30% of terminal cancer patients, nausea in more than 50%, and both can lead to significant morbidity.

Many patients fear the nausea and vomiting associated with cancer treatments. The introduction of newer anti-emetics has radically altered the effectiveness of the management of these symptoms.

Mechanism

The vomiting centre, located in the lateral reticular formation of the medulla, is an area which when stimulated leads to vomiting. Efferent pathways from the vomiting centre co-ordinate the vomiting response, leading to effects such as salivation, gastric relaxation and abdominal muscle contraction.

Afferent signals to the vomiting centre are received from a variety of sources. These include:

- The chemoreceptor trigger zone (CTZ), located in the medulla, is a region sensitive to chemical stimuli, such as chemotherapeutic agents. With no blood–brain barrier in this region of the brain, the CTZ is able to sample both cerebrospinal fluid and blood directly. Chemotherapy is believed to lead to the release of neurotransmitters (see below) from sensitive cells damaged by the drug.
- The visceral organs, a variety of receptors such as chemoreceptors, nocioreceptors and mechano-receptors, trigger afferent pathways which pass via the vagal and sympathetic nerves and stimulate the vomiting centre.
- The vestibular-labyrinthine apparatus of the inner ear, in response to body motion.
- Higher centres in response to sensory stimulation such as smell and taste, psychological distress and pain.

Neurotransmitters

Peripheral neuroreceptors and the CTZ are known to contain receptors for a variety of neurotransmitters. The afferent pathways to the vomiting centre are mediated by several neurotransmitters and their specific receptors. These include:

- Dopamine (D_2) receptor. These are present in high numbers in the chemoreceptor trigger zone.
- Serotonin (5-hydroxytryptamine, $5\text{-}HT_3$) receptor. $5\text{-}HT_3$ receptors are present throughout the CNS, especially in those areas receiving afferents from the GI tract.
- Histamine and acetylcholine receptors.
- Opiate receptors.

This explains the diversity of pharmacological agents employed to treat emesis.

Causes

The causes of nausea and vomiting in cancer patients are diverse. These include:

1. Physical complications of cancer (e.g. obstruction from GI tumours, extrinsic compression by intra-abdominal disease or increased intra-cranial pressure from brain metastases).

2. Drug induced. Antibiotics and the gastric irritation from NSAIDs may cause drug-induced emesis. However, the most severe symptoms often relate to the cytotoxic chemotherapy itself.

The severity of nausea and vomiting is associated with:

- Drug used. Cisplatin, DTIC and cyclophosphamide are associated with some degree of nausea and vomiting in up to 90% of individuals, which may be severe without appropriate treatment. Carboplatin, CCNU, doxorubicin and etoposide are associated with nausea and vomiting to a lesser degree. Drugs such as 5-FU, methotrexate, vincristine and vinblastine are rarely associated with severe emesis.
- Drug schedule. Both the dose and speed of administration may affect the degree of nausea and vomiting. Combination chemotherapy may lead to greater nausea and vomiting than that associated with each agent individually.
- Other factors. Women are generally affected more than men. A history of previous heavy alcohol consumption reduces the risk.

Delayed emesis is defined as nausea or vomiting occurring more than 24 hours following chemotherapy administration. It occurs most frequently in patients receiving cisplatin and, generally occurs 48–72 hours following the drug and may be experienced by up to 60% of patients.

3. Metabolic complications (e.g. hypercalcaemia and uraemia).

4. Radiation induced. radiation of the brain or abdomen may lead to emesis.

5. Psychological. Anticipatory vomiting precedes the administration of chemotherapy and often occurs in response to a trigger, such as entering the hospital. It is a learned response conditioned by the severity and duration of previous emesis.

Management

A variety of techniques may be employed to control nausea and vomiting. Anti-emetic drugs may be effective in controlling the symptoms of most patients but alternative strategies may be required depending on the cause of the symptoms.

Drug therapy

Anti-emetics may be given orally, intravenously, subcutaneously or rectally. Oral medication is inappropriate with active vomiting and parenteral administration is required. Subcutanous administration via a syringe driver is often effective, providing constant systemic administration of appropriate antiemetics (e.g. cyclizine and haloperidol).

Anti-emetics are used prophylactically to prevent the nausea and vomiting associated with chemotherapy.

Single-agent anti-emetics may be effective, but combinations of drugs which act in different ways are used frequently, especially in the management of chemotherapy-induced emesis.

Many of the drugs employed act by inhibition of specific neurotransmitter receptors.

1. Dopamine antagonists. These are the most commonly used anti-emetic agents. At standard doses these drugs are not effective with highly emetogenic drugs (e.g. cisplatin-induced vomiting). High-dose therapy reduces the severity of cisplatin-induced vomiting but anti-dopaminergic effects limit its use. A range of different dopamine antagonists are employed.

- Metoclopramide. This is the most frequently prescribed anti-emetic in the management of chemotherapy-induced nausea and vomiting.
- Butyrophenones (e.g. haloperidol).
- Phenothiazines (e.g. prochlorperazine).
- Domperidone.

2. *5-HT$_3$ antagonists.* The introduction of the 5-HT$_3$ receptor antagonists such as ondansetron and granisetron has significantly affected the morbidity associated with highly emetogenic chemotherapy such as cisplatin. Prior to their introduction, first-dose cisplatin was associated with a median of 12 vomiting episodes in the first 24 hours; with 5-HT$_3$ administration 50% of patients now experience no vomiting. 5-HT$_3$ antagonists are no more effective in managing delayed vomiting than other antiemetics. The side effects of the 5-HT$_3$ antagonists are uncommon but may include headache, light-headedness, diarrhoea and skin rashes.

3. *Corticosteroids* (e.g. dexamethasone). These are frequently employed as an adjunct to other anti-emetic drugs. The mode of action in preventing emesis is, however, unclear. It may be associated with hyperglycaemia and psychotic reactions particularly in the elderly.

4. *Others.* These include:

- Anti-histamines (e.g. cyclizine), can be a useful alternative to dopamine antagonists.
- Benzodiazepines (e.g. lorazepam), have minimal anti-emetic effect but their anxiolytic, sedative and amnesic properties are useful in anticipatory vomiting.
- Cannabinoids (e.g. nabilone). Nabilone, a cannabis derivative, is licensed for the management of

chemotherapy-induced nausea and vomiting in patients resistant to standard therapy.

Surgery   Surgical intervention may be the most effective method of achieving symptom control where emesis is due to mechanical obstruction and may even be justified in end stage disease.

Radiotherapy   Cerebral metastases may be managed with radiotherapy in combination with corticosteroids.

Psychological   Psychological support including specific counselling techniques such as neurolinguistic reprogramming may be effective in patients in whom there is a psychological element. Some patients derive benefit from the use of alternative therapies such as the 'Sea-band'.

Current issues

New drugs   New drugs with combined 5-HT_3 antagonistic and 5-HT_4 agonist activity are being evaluated in clinical trials.

Further reading

Roila F, Favero A. Antiemetics revisited. *Current Opinion in Oncology,* 1997; 321–6.

Related topics of interest

Chemotherapy – (d) complications (p. 58)
Palliative care (p. 194)

NON-HODGKIN'S LYMPHOMA

Non-Hodgkin's lymphomas (NHL) are derived from clonal proliferations of lymphocytes or their developmental precursors. Most are derived from B-lymphocytes, but T-cell lymphomas are an important and clinically complex group. The NHLs represent a heterogeneous group of malignancies with differing patterns of clinical behaviour and response to treatment.

Background

Incidence

Approximately 7000 cases of NHL are diagnosed annually in the UK with more than 4000 NHL-related deaths. It is predominantly a disease of late middle age with a median age of approximately 55 years. The incidence of NHL is rising, with an increase world-wide of 150% since the 1950s.

Aetiology

1. *Chromosomal abnormalities.* Cytogenetic abnormalities can be identified in more than 85% of NHL. Specific NHLs are associated with specific chromosomal translocations. The 14:18 translocation is associated with follicular B-cell lymphoma which leads to overexpression of *bcl-2*.

2. *Viruses.* The Epstein–Barr virus (EBV) has been identified in Burkitt's lymphoma cells. The human T-cell leukaemia virus type 1 (HTLV-1) is associated with an aggressive T-cell lymphoma.

3. *Immunosuppression.* Immunodeficiency, both primary and acquired, are associated with an increased incidence of NHL. EBV and other viral infections have a role in their pathogenesis and these are usually diffuse B-cell lymphomas.

4. *Helicobacter pylori.* Mucosal-associated lymphoid tissue (MALT) lymphoma is associated with the presence of *Helicobacter pylori* in the stomach.

5. *Coeliac disease.* This is associated with an increased incidence of T-cell lymphomas of the intestine.

Histology	The NHLs are a diverse group of neoplasms with distinct behaviours. Histological classifications have been designed to identify distinct sub-groups in an attempt to predict prognosis and guide treatment.

The NHLs are a diverse group of neoplasms with distinct behaviours. Histological classifications have been designed to identify distinct sub-groups in an attempt to predict prognosis and guide treatment.

There are a variety of systems by which the NHLs are classified. These include the Rappaport classification, the Kiel classification, the Working formulation, and most recently the REAL (revised European–American lymphoma) classification. The continuing development of new schemes reflects the advances in diagnostic techniques such as immunohistochemistry and cytogenetics and their ability to distinguish between different NHLs with distinct clinical behaviours.

The REAL classification attempts to classify lymphomas by cell of origin, that is B-cell neoplasms, T/NK cell neoplasms (and Hodgkin's disease).

Clinical features

Presentation

NHL usually arises in peripheral nodes and presents as a painless enlargement of a lymph node. Symptoms may relate to compression of surrounding tissues by the enlarging nodes. Up to 50% present at an extranodal site, such as the stomach, intestine, bone, CNS, lung, thyroid, testis and skin. Weight loss, night sweats, fever and pruritis may occur.

Investigation

Biopsy is mandatory to enable an accurate diagnosis through conventional histology and immuno-phenotyping. Staging investigations also include CT of the chest, abdomen and pelvis, bone-marrow aspirate and trephine, lumbar puncture and CSF cytospin analysis. Serum LDH provides prognostic information.

Staging

NHL is most frequently staged with the Ann Arbor classification, although the predictive value of this classification is less clear than for Hodgkin's disease.

Stage I: involvement of a single lymph node region or a lymphoid structure.

Stage II: two or more lymph node regions or structures on one side of the diaphragm.

Stage III: involvement of lymph node regions or structures on both sides of the diaphragm.

Stage IV: disseminated involvement of extralymphatic organs with or without lymph nodes.

Each stage is further classified by the absence (A) or presence (B) of 'B' symptoms: weight loss (>10%), fever and drenching night sweats.

Management

NHL is generally sensitive to both chemotherapy and radiotherapy.

Surgery

The main role of surgery is in establishing the diagnosis with an excision node biopsy or tissue biopsy. Surgery may rarely be used as the primary treatment modality, for example advanced gastric lymphoma.

Radiotherapy

Radiotherapy may be curative in localized low-grade lymphoma with more than 50% of patients disease-free 10 years later. However, such a presentation is infrequent. Localized intermediate and high-grade lymphoma may be treated with involved field radiotherapy with some cures, but frequently the addition of combination chemotherapy is needed.

Chemotherapy

1. Low grade. Disseminated disease is rarely cured with chemotherapy. Symptomatic patients can be treated with single-agent chemotherapy, such as oral chlorambucil. Combination chemotherapy regimes may achieve remissions of longer duration. However, no survival benefit has been demonstrated.

2. Intermediate and high grade. Combination chemotherapy may be curative for patients with intermediate and high-grade NHL. No single regimen has been demonstrated to have superior efficacy. CHOP (cyclophosphamide/doxorubicin/vincristine/prednisolone) remains the most frequently used, although other regimens are also used. Complete response rates are up to 80%, with cure rates of 30–40%.

3. High-dose chemotherapy. Randomized controlled studies have shown a benefit for high-dose chemotherapy in the management of certain lymphoma patients. It is currently employed in the management of relapse, primary resistant disease and those patients with bad prognostic factors at presentation.

Immunotherapy

1.   Interferon-α. Up to 40% of patients with low-grade NHL respond to interferon-α with 10–15% achieving a complete remission. It has been demonstrated to improve survival in follicular NHL.

Antibiotics

MALT lymphoma of the stomach associated with *Helicobacter pylori* may resolve following eradication of the organism with appropriate antibiotics.

Prognostic factors

Histology

1.   Low grade. Most patients will have prolonged survival but ultimately die from their disease. However, the median survival is 7–8 years.

2.   High and intermediate grade. About one third of patients are cured.

Shipp index

Multivariate analysis has demonstrated a number of factors to predict prognosis in patients with high-grade lymphoma. The same factors are also applicable to low-grade disease. The factors associated with a poor prognosis are:

- Age: greater than 60.
- Serum LDH: above normal range.
- Performance status: 2 or more.
- Stage 3 or 4 disease.
- Extranodal involvement at more than one site.

Current issues

Monoclonal antibodies

These are antibodies targeted to antigens expressed on the surface of malignant lymphocytes. Antibodies have been conjugated to toxins such as ricin and saporin or to radionuclides.

High-dose chemotherapy

The role of high-dose chemotherapy in low-grade lymphoma is being evaluated.

| Improved diagnostics | The use of molecular biology techniques, such as the polymerase chain reaction (see Polymerase chain reaction), to detect specific genetic markers, such as translocations, has been applied to both the inital diagnosis and the detection of minimal residual disease post-therapy. |

Further reading

DeVita VT, Jr. In: DeVita VT, Jr, Hellman S, Rosenburg SA, eds. *Cancer Principles and Practice of Oncology.* Philadelphia: Lippincott-Raven, 1997; 44.3.

Harris NL, Jaffe ES, Stein H *et al.* A revised European–American classification of lymphoid neoplasms: a proposal from the International Lymphoma Study Group. *Blood,* 1994; **84:** 1361–92.

Shipp M. Prognostic factors in aggressive non-Hodgkin's lymphoma: who has high risk disease? *Blood,* 1994; **83:** 1165–73.

Related topics of interest

OESOPHAGEAL CANCER

Incidence

The incidence and mortality of carcinoma of the oesophagus are both approximately 5000 cases per year reflecting the poor prognosis associated with the disease. Peak incidence is between 60 and 80 years of age. Overall, there is a male predominance with a ratio of 3:2.

Aetiology

The aetiology of carcinoma of the oesophagus is unknown. Tobacco and alcohol use are both strongly related and demonstrate a dose-related effect. Only one in eight patients with carcinoma of the oesophagus neither smoke nor drink alcohol. World-wide, dietary factors are important.

Barrett's oesophagus, glandular metaplasia arising in the squamous epithelium of the distal third of the oesophagus as a result of chronic gastro-oesophageal reflux, is strongly associated with adenocarcinoma of the oesophagus (30- to 40-fold increased risk) and is therefore considered a pre-malignant condition. Benign oesophageal strictures, achlasia, Plummer–Vinson syndrome, tylosis, syphilis and repeated oral infections are all associated with an increased risk.

Histology

Tumours may arise at any point within the oesophagus. However, less than 10% arise in the upper third, 35–40% in the middle third and 40–45% in the lower third. The histological types seen are:

1. *Squamous cell.* These comprise more than 80% of all malignant tumours. They account for almost all of the tumours arising in the upper two thirds of the oesophagus.

2. *Adenocarcinoma.* These used to account for less than 5% of all oesophageal carcinoma. Their incidence is rising and with a decrease in overall incidence, account for up to 35% of all tumours in some series. Adenocarcinomas arise principally in the distal oesophagus. They are strongly associated with Barrett's oesophagus (59–86% of all cases).

3. Others. Rare histological types in oesophageal tumours include small cell, melanoma, carcinoid and leiomyosarcoma.

Local spread of oesophageal cancer occurs both circumferentially and longitudinally. Lymphatic spread occurs early, about two thirds of cases involving lymph nodes by the time of diagnosis. Haematogenous spread, via the portal vein, principally involves the liver. Other common sites of metastases include lungs, bone and brain.

Clinical features

Presentation

The most common symptom in oesophageal cancer is dysphagia, with or without regurgitation. Regurgitation may result in aspiration and subsequent pneumonia. Pneumonia may also result from oesophago-tracheal and oesophago-bronchial fistulae, caused by local spread of the tumour. Significant weight loss (>10%) and malnutrition are also common presenting features. Recurrent laryngeal nerve palsy may occur. Upper GI bleeding, presenting as haematemesis or melaena, is rare in oesophageal cancer. Pain, usually retro-sternal, usually occurs late.

Investigations

Upper GI endoscopy. This is the investigation of choice as biopsy and/or brushings for cytology may be obtained.

Trans-oesophageal ultrasound. This may further delineate the degree of mucosal invasion.

CT. CT is central to the assessment of stage, which helps to define and appropriate management plan. It is particularly useful for assessing the spread to mediastinal lymph nodes.

Staging

The TNM classification for oesophageal carcinoma is as follows:

Tx   Primary tumour cannot be assessed.
T0   No evidence of primary tumour.

Tis	Carcinoma *in situ.*
Ta	Non-invasive papillary tumour.
T1	Tumour invades lamina propria or submucosa.
T2	Tumour invades muscularis mucosa.
T3	Tumour invades adventitia.
T4	Tumour invades adjacent structures.
N0	No evidence of regional lymph nodes.
N1	Regional lymph node metastases.
M0	No distant metastases.
M1	Distant metastases present.

Management

Many patients with oesophageal carcinoma present with advanced disease and the focus of their management is therefore palliative.

Surgery

Surgical resection of the tumour is performed using a wide variety of techniques, usually with combined thoracotomy and laparotomy. Curative resection is generally only appropriate in patients with a good performance status, good nutritional state and in whom there is no evidence of metastatic disease. Local lymph nodes may be resected at the time of operation. A recent review of oesophageal resection suggested that 56% of patients have resectable disease, but 12.5% of those operated die from post-operative complications.

Bypass procedures may be performed and frequently achieve good palliation of dysphagia. However, an operative mortality of 20–30% occurs. Dilatation of an obstructing lesion or insertion of a semi-rigid tube, for example a Celestin tube, may also relieve dysphagia.

Radiotherapy

Radiotherapy may be administered via external beam or intra-luminal brachytherapy via a naso-gastric tube.

Radical radiotherapy (50–65 Gy fractionated over 4–6 weeks) may be given with curative intent. Upper third tumours are frequently managed in this way due to the complexity of surgery. Five year survival rates for patients treated in this way range are approximately 5%.

Radiotherapy may also be used as an adjunct to surgical resection, either neoadjuvantly in an attempt to downstage the tumour prior to resection or post-operatively to improve the outcome following resection. However, there is no clear evidence that adjuvant or neo-adjuvant radiotherapy produces an overall survival benefit compared with surgery alone.

Palliative radiotherapy (40–50 Gy) may be used to treat dysphagia and/or pain in patients in whom curative treatment is not possible.

Chemotherapy

Chemotherapy has generally been used in patients with advanced disease. Single-agent chemotherapy, in common with most solid tumours, produces few responses. Combination therapy with drugs such as cisplatin and 5-FU improve response rates although such responses are generally short-lived. The role of chemotherapy in combination with other treatment modalities in a neoadjuvant or adjuvant manner is the focus of current research.

Prognostic factors

Overall prognosis in oesophageal cancer is poor, with 5 year survival rates of only 5–10%. Prognosis is related to stage of disease at presentation. Following surgical resection, survival rates at 1, 3 and 5 years were reported as 55, 25 and 20%, respectively.

Screening/prevention

Knowledge of the aetiological agents in oesophageal cancer provides the opportunity for prevention via health education, for example advice to stop smoking and reduce alcohol consumption. The identification of Barrett's oesophagus as a pre-malignant condition allows for monitoring by annual endoscopy. The role of prophylactic excision of areas of metaplasia is controversial

Current issues

These include neo-adjuvant chemotherapy.

Further reading

Peracchia A *et al*. In: Peckham M, Pinedo H, Veroneri U, eds. *Oxford Textbook of Oncology*, Oxford University Press, 1995; 1983–2052.

OVARIAN CANCER

Background

Incidence

Over 5000 new cases of ovarian carcinoma are diagnosed in the UK each year. The annual incidence rate is 177 cases per million women and it is therefore the fifth commonest cancer in women in the UK. Ninety per cent of cases occur after the age of 45 years, over half of all cases occur in women over the age of 65.

Risk factors

Increased. Infertility, late menopause and family history. Family history is especially important if there are greater than two first-degree relatives with ovarian carcinoma. Familial predisposition is also seen in families with mutations of the *BRCA1* gene and the more recently characterized *BRCA2* gene. These families have a greater risk of both ovarian and breast cancer.

Decreased. Increasing numbers of pregnancies, use of oral contraceptives.

Aetiology

Several pathogenic processes have been proposed for ovarian carcinoma. The epithelial lining of the ovary requires constant remodelling following ovulation and this predisposes to malignant change. Inclusion cysts occurring due to implantation of epithelial cells into the stroma at the time of ovulation may also lead to malignant change.

Ovarian carcinoma spreads by local shedding of cells into the peritoneal cavity with implantation of peritoneal surfaces. Lymphatic and haematogenous spread also occur.

Histology

- Epithelial cell. Originate from the surface of the ovary (90% of tumours).
- (a) Serous cystadenocarcinoma.
- (b) Mucinous cystadenocarcinoma.
- (c) Endometroid adenocarcinomas.
- (d) Clear cell adenocarcinomas.
- (e) Undifferentiated adenocarcinomas.

- Germ cell. Arise from the ovarian cortex (1–2% of tumours).
- Ovarian sarcomas.
- Granulosa cell tumours.

Clinical features

Presentation

Early ovarian carcinoma is often asymptomatic and therefore presents at a late stage. Vague symptoms include abdominal distension, pain nausea and vomiting, bowel disturbance and occasionally vaginal bleeding. Ascites is generally a late feature and is thought to be due to blockage of the draining lymphatics.

Investigations

CA125. A serum level greater than 200 U/ml is highly suggestive of ovarian malignancy. The level at baseline has no prognostic significance but after three cycles of chemotherapy its level (and its decline) correlates highly with survival.

Ultrasound. The first-line investigation for the detection of an ovarian mass. Trans-vaginal ultrasound is more sensitive than routine abdominal imaging. The assessment of ovarian artery blood flow using colour flow Doppler, can be used to distinguish benign from malignant ovarian masses.

CT. Advanced ovarian carcinoma has a highly characteristic CT appearance. The disease is often confined within the peritoneal cavity, with pelvic masses, omental disease and serosal metastases of bowel, liver, spleen and diaphragms.

Pleural fluid cytology. Pleural effusions are common in advanced ovarian carcinoma. The distinction between 'reactive' and malignant effusions is important because it differentiates stage 3c and 4 disease (see below).

Staging

The most commonly used classification is that of FIGO (International Federation of Gynaecology and Obstetrics).
Stage 1:   growth limited to the ovaries.

1A:	one ovary.
1B:	both ovaries.
1C:	1A or 1B and malignant ascites, positive peritoneal washings, surface disease or capsule rupture.

Stage 2:   growth involving one or both ovaries with pelvic spread.

2A:	extension to adnexae (Fallopian tubes and uterus).
2B:	extension to other pelvic tissues.
2C:	2A or 2b and malignant cells in ascites or peritoneal washings or capsule rupture.

Stage 3:   tumour involvement of abdominal cavity.

3A:	microscopic peritoneal metastasis beyond pelvis
3B:	macroscopic peritoneal metastasis <2 cm.
3C:	peritoneal metastasis >2 cm and/or involvement of retroperitoneal or inguinal lymph nodes.

Stage 4:   distant metastases. Commonly lung (malignant pleural effusion) or liver (parenchymal, rather than serosal). Other sites of metastatic disease, brain, bone are unusual.

Management

Surgery

The role of maximal debulking surgery is well established. Total abdominal hysterectomy, bilateral salpingo-oophorectomy, omentectomy and multiple peritoneal biopsies should be performed through a vertical incision by a surgeon specializing in oncological gynaecology. This enables a full inspection of the abdominal cavity so the amount of residual disease can be accurately assessed. This has both prognostic and therapeutic implications. A second look laparotomy is the most sensitive way to assess disease response but is rarely performed today. Chemotherapy may enable optimal debulking surgery in patients previously considered inoperable or suboptimally debulked but this remains a research area.

Chemotherapy

Ovarian carcinoma is relatively sensitive to chemotherapy and therefore should be used routinely, even for advanced stage 4 disease. However, in patients with good prognosis Stage 1 disease chemotherapy may not be required.

Drugs with high activity in ovarian carcinoma are the platinum drugs (cisplatin and carboplatin), alkylating agents (cyclophosphamide), anthracyclines (doxorubucin) and the taxanes (Taxol and Taxotere).

First-line chemotherapy is with platinum-based drugs (i.e. cisplatin or carboplatin), either as single agents or in combination with alkylating agents +/- anthracyclines. Response rates of 50–70% are obtained with these strategies. The use of Taxol in combination with platinum drugs is currently being investigated in randomized clinical trials. Response rates are similar to those obtained with platinum drugs.

Second-line chemotherapy is given in two contexts. Platinum-resistant disease has been shown to respond to Taxol in about 20% of cases. Patients with platinum-sensitive disease, who relapse more than 6 months following such chemotherapy may benefit from rechallenge cisplatin or carboplatin (response rate approx. 30%)

Tamoxifen (20 mg bd) has been shown to have an effect in approximately 20% of disease resistant to other chemotherapeutic agents. This treatment is well tolerated in patients with a poor performance status. Chronic low-dose oral etoposide has a similar level of activity in this setting.

Radiotherapy

Total abdominal radiotherapy has been used in the past. The side effects include gastrointestinal dysfunction and subacute bowel obstruction and its use is declining.

Prognostic factors

Stage of tumour

Stage 1: 70%   5 year survival.
Stage 2: 50%   5 year survival.
Stage 3: 20%   5 year survival.
Stage 4: 4%   5 year survival.

Histology	Cell type and degree of differentiation of the tumour affect prognosis.
Residual disease	The volume of residual disease post surgery directly relates to both response rate and survival. This may reflect surgical skill but the biology of the disease is also important.
Performance status	A worse performance status is associated with a poorer prognosis.

Screening

Abdominal ultrasound and CA125 can detect ovarian pathology but is not sufficiently specific to be used in the general population. However, investigation continues particularly in high-risk families. Several large ongoing studies are investigating the use of CA125, other tumour markers and trans-vaginal ultrasound to screen post-menopausal women.

Current issues

The current International Collaborative Ovarian Neoplasm study (ICON 2) compares combination therapy (cisplatin, adriamycin and cyclophosphamide; CAP) with full-dose single-agent carboplatin. This will resolve which of these established regimes is the optimum first-line chemotherapy. The ICON 3 trial will extend this by comparing first-line CAP or carboplatin to Taxol and carboplatin. This will determine whether a Taxol-containing combination therapy, as initial treatment, is more effective than current regimes.

The role of intraperitoneal chemotherapy and IFNα to maintain remission achieved by standard chemotherapy, are both currently under evaluation.

Screening is of current interest for detecting familial cases. Improving survival outcomes with chemotherapy is under evaluation.

PAEDIATRIC ONCOLOGY

Paediatric oncologists manage a wide spectrum of cancers which is very different from that seen in adults. Many children's cancers are derived from embryonic tissues. At diagnosis, the disease is usually disseminated and generally responds well to treatment, with a much better overall outcome than in adults. Epithelial carcinomas (most commonly thyroid and nasopharyngeal) are extremely rare in children (<2%).

Background

Incidence

In the paediatric population (defined as those less than 15 years old) cancer is rare. In the UK child population of 12.5 million, only 1200 new cases occur each year. However, malignancy is the second commonest cause of death in the 1–15 year-old age group (behind accidents), accounting for 14% of deaths.

Aetiology

The causes of childhood cancer are essentially unknown. The effect of environmental carcinogens is small due to a short exposure time, and that of the ageing process negligible. Inherent host factors are more significant.

Genetic factors

1. *Inherited.*

- Mendelian inherited conditions, e.g. neurofibromatosis.
- Fragile chromosome syndromes with defective DNA repair, e.g. ataxia telangiectasia.
- Immunodeficiency syndromes, e.g. Wiscott–Aldrich.
- Li–Fraumeni syndrome.

2. *Non-inherited.*

- Point deletions, for example retinoblastoma.
- Chromosomal abnormalities, for example Down's syndrome.

Viruses

1. *Epstein–Barr.* This infection is associated with B-cell lymphoid malignancies and nasopharyngeal carcinoma.

2. *HIV.* This infection is associated with lymphoma

and Kaposi's sarcoma.

Ionizing radiation

Prenatal exposure to diagnostic X-rays leads to a 1.5-fold increase in leukaemia incidence.

Postnatal exposure increases the risk of some tumours such as thyroid cancer. Secondary tumours can occur within therapeutic radiation fields.

Drugs

1. Prenatal exposure. Maternal ingestion of diethylstilboestrol, for example, is associated with vaginal clear cell carcinoma in the female offspring many years later.

2. Immunosuppressive drugs. For example, a reported 20–40% increased risk of lymphoma with the intense immunosuppressive regime following renal transplantation is believed to be linked to defective immunosurveillance.

3. Cytotoxic drugs. Secondary malignancies may follow treatment with cytotoxic chemotherapy.

Histology

The spectrum of malignancies is different to that seen with adults. The relative incidence of paediatric malignancies is as follows:

Leukaemia	35%	(80% ALL)
CNS	20%	
Lymphoma	15%	
Solid tumours		
Embryonic	15%	neuroblastoma
		nephroblastoma
		retinoblastoma
Sarcomas	12%	rhabdomyosarcoma
		osteosarcoma
		Ewing's sarcoma
Others	3%	

Management

The management of all children with cancer should be based in a specialist treatment centre as survival is improved relative to non-specialist centres. In the UK this is predominantly in United Kingdom Children's Cancer Study Group (UKCCSG) centres.

Assessment	In patients with a suspicion of malignant disease, referral to a specialist centre before biopsy is preferable. This allows modern diagnostic techniques, such as cytogenetic and molecular investigations, to be performed on fresh tissue. The biopsy performed needs to be carefully considered with respect to future surgical treatment.
Treatment	Most children with cancer in the UK are treated in multi-centre collaborative clinical trials, co-ordinated mainly by the UKCCSG, but also by MRC or European study groups. The numbers treated by individual centres are too small to allow local studies. Results are continually evaluated to enable treatment to be modified and protocols revised.
	Long-term survival following paediatric malignancy has been greatly improved following the introduction of combination chemotherapy regimes. Most paediatric malignancies are now managed with complex combinations of chemotherapy (often with additional surgery and radiotherapy).
Supportive care	A co-ordinated multidisciplinary team approach is utilized which includes medical and technological services, nursing care and psychosocial support. Nutritional, educational and developmental aspects of care are also areas of vital importance to paediatric patients.
	Care is family centred. Social and psychological support is provided for parents and siblings as well as the affected child.

Prognostic factors and survival

The improved outlook for the child with cancer can be considered among the major advances in both oncology and paediatrics of the last 30 years. The overall incidence of cancer has remained stable but survival and quality of life have greatly improved.

The overall survival rate is now 65%. However, this varies with tumour type, site and extent of spread. Some tumours still have an extremely poor outlook.

Five year survival rates (%)

Year of diagnosis:	1954–63	1964–73	1974–83	1986–89
Overall	21	34	49	65
ALL	2	20	60	70
Retinoblastoma	84	85	87	86
Wilms tumour	31	59	80	80
Ewing's sarcoma	9	14	41	60
Medulloblastoma	–	35	45	45
Osteosarcoma	15	15	25	60

Factors improving survival
- Improved supportive care, e.g. transfusion support, better treatment of infective complications, nutritional supplementation, prevention of adverse drug effects, use of central venous catheters, development of paediatric ICUs and specialist paediatric oncology nursing care.
- Care in UKCCSG centres.
- Enrolment in collaborative clinical trials.
- Multidisciplinary collaboration.
- Screening: pre-symptomatic screening of family members and syndromic cases.

Late effects

By the year 2000, one in 1000 20-year-olds will be survivors from childhood cancer. Long-term sequelae of treatment and their effects on quality of life are therefore of paramount importance.

Long-term follow up services are required to detect potential problems which may result from the primary disease or its complications, delayed effects of surgery, radiotherapy or chemotherapy, and from psychosocial problems consequent upon the illness or treatment.

Side effects

1. Impaired growth. This may result from endocrine dysfunction, steroid toxicity, or a direct effect on bone and soft tissues by radiotherapy, especially during periods of rapid growth.

2. Impaired development. Radiotherapy is known to affect the maturing brain and is therefore used cautiously in young children with ALL and brain tumours.

3. *Endocrine abnormalities*. Cranial radiation can cause pituitary dysfunction. The thyroid gland is also vulnerable to radiation.

4. *Infertility*. Many cytotoxic agents, particularly alkylating agents, lead to infertility.

5. *Organ damage*. Toxicity to specific organs such as the heart, lungs or kidneys may become relevant as the patient ages.

6. *Psychological*. Emotional and social consequences of aggressive therapy may occur especially if there are severe deformities or limited vital organ function.

7. *Secondary tumours*. Incidence estimations range from 5.6–12% at 25 years from diagnosis. This is 10–20 times the risk of cancer in the general population of age-matched controls. Whether genetic pre-disposition or carcinogenic effect of treatment is to blame is unresolved.

8. *Effect on future offspring*. This has recently been investigated and is thought to be negligible.

Current issues

Molecular biology

Advances in the molecular characterization of childhood cancers has delineated several gene defects, for example the retinoblastoma (*Rb*) oncogene. Such molecular changes are being assessed as prognostic markers.

New treatments

The role of intensive chemotherapy regimens in poor prognosis patients is being assessed.

Further reading

Paediatric tumours. In: Peckham M, Pinedo H, Veroneri U, eds. *Oxford Textbook of Oncology*. Oxford University Press, 1995; 1983–2052.

PAIN CONTROL IN CANCER

Studies in the UK indicate that 25–50% of cancer patients experience pain at diagnosis rising to 75% with advanced disease. Most doctors should be able to provide pain control following the WHO guidelines in more than 80% of cancer patients with pain. In more difficult situations help can be sought from hospital palliative care teams, a local hospice or consultant in pain management (usually an anaesthetist).

Objectives　　Complete relief from pain can be achieved rapidly in some patients but for the majority, some degree of control is the first goal. This is easiest to achieve at night and at rest and hardest to control on movement. It is important to set realistic targets with the patient to help them to cope with the pain. This prevents loss of confidence by the patient if immediate and sustained relief from pain is expected by them which may not be possible.

Classification　　Pain may be classified as:

- Nociceptive: pain of visceral, soft tissue or bone origin.
- Neuropathic: pain due to pressure on or damage to nerves. A neuropathic origin is likely when pain is experienced in an area of altered sensation.

Assessment　　Up to 80% of cancer patients have more than one discrete pain and 30% have four or more. A careful history and examination of each pain is important if pain control is to be achieved.

Radiological or electrophysiological investigations can provide useful information if the pain origin cannot be determined. The patients' psychological state should be assessed with regard to depression, social, financial or spiritual worries, all of which can make pain more difficult to cope with and harder to control.

After the diagnosis has been made and treatment started, a vital aspect of successful pain management is frequent review.

Management

Control of the underlying disease process by surgery, chemotherapy or radiotherapy is the ideal form of pain management. However, additional methods are indicated concurrently or when primary anti-cancer treatment is ineffective or not indicated.

| Analgesic ladder | The WHO analgesic ladder recommends commencing treatment with NSAIDs or paracetamol. If the pain persists or increases despite optimal doses, the drugs should be changed to weak opioids such as codeine or DF118 (i.e. the next rung on the ladder). The use of strong opioids (e.g. morphine, diamorphine, fentanyl) should be the next progression if pain control is inadequate. |

The WHO ladder also emphasizes the need to consider alternative drugs with indirect analgesic activity (i.e. adjuvant drugs).

Adjuvant drugs

Adjuvant drugs have a co-analgesic effect and may decrease the need for higher doses of standard analgesics.

- Pain related to an inflammatory reaction may respond to the use of steroids such as oral dexamethasone.
- Drugs such as tricyclic antidepressants (e.g. amitriptyline) or anticonvulsants (e.g. sodium valproate) are of particular use in neuropathic pain.
- Anti-arryhthmic drugs, such as mexiletine or flecainide, and subcutaneous ketamine are occasionally used but require specialist advice.
- Bone pain unresponsive to radiotherapy and NSAIDs may sometimes respond to intravenous bisphosphonates using similar doses as those used to treat hypercalcaemia.

Anaesthetic techniques

Nerve blocks using steroid and local anaesthetic can provide good pain control in selected patients. The most commonly used are coeliac plexus block, intercostal block or paravertebral blocks.

Epidural or intrathecal infusions of opioids with local anaesthetic drugs can provide excellent pain control when standard routes of administration have failed or side effects limit dose escalation. Spinal administration of drugs allow higher concentrations of opioids to be achieved in the dorsal horn and periaquaductal grey areas of the CNS than with systemic administration. In addition, blockade of nerve roots or spinal cord with local anaesthetic may be the only option in controlling pain from a bone fracture or extensive tissue damage caused by tumour.

Surgical techniques	Orthopaedic referral may be indicated if mechanical instability is the cause of pain.
Non-drug methods	The following are often available from physiotherapists, pain teams or palliative care teams:

- Transcutaneous nerve stimulation (TENS).
- Acupuncture.
- Physiotherapy.
- Aromatherapy.

Psychological approaches	Some cancer patients benefit from cognitive or behavioural approaches for their pain management. In many patients, acknowledging and treating underlying depression and addressing other concerns should be part of a multifaceted approach when controlling their pain.

Related topic of interest

Morphine (p. 155)
Palliative care (p. 194)

PALLIATIVE CARE

Definitions

1. Palliative care (World Health Organisation). The active, total care of patients whose disease is incurable. Its goal is the achievement of the best possible quality of life for patients and their families. Control of physical, psychosocial and spiritual problems is paramount. Palliative care affirms life and regards dying as a normal process, it neither hastens nor postpones death.

2. Palliative medicine (Association for Palliative Medicine). The study and management of patients with active, progressive, far advanced disease for whom the prognosis is limited and the focus of care is the quality of life. Palliative medicine has been recognized as a separate medical speciality since 1987.

Objectives

The Royal College of Physicians has issued guidelines on the characteristics of good palliative care which include:

- Attention to the whole needs of the individual.
- Relief of symptoms.
- Care extending beyond patients to families.
- Emphasis on quality of life.
- Good communication.
- Strong multi-disciplinary teamwork.

The process

Specialized and generalized care. Due to the demands on the services, a distinction is increasingly made between generalized and specialized palliative care.

Generalized palliative care is within the scope of all doctors and nurses and involves attentive listening, basic symptom control (usually through disease control rather than cure) and a clear commitment to the patient's quality of life. Patients with incurable illnesses who require mainly nursing care may be more appropriately managed in a nursing home rather than a hospice if they cannot be cared for at home.

Specialized palliative care concentrates on control of difficult physical and psychological symptoms coupled with practical and emotional support for patients and their families. Many units offer bereavement services for carers with complicated grief.

Service organization. In order to meet its objectives, specialist palliative care services are organized to meet the needs of patients in a variety of clinical settings. At home, the patient's general practitioner and district nurse form the primary care team and are advised by palliative home care teams. These teams are usually attached to a local hospice but may be linked to a local health centre. They consist of experienced nurses funded either by a major charity (e.g. Cancer Relief Macmillan Fund or Marie Curie Foundation), a district health authority or local hospice. Some have community-based consultants working with them. These teams advise on symptom control and can provide psychosocial support for the patient and family. If the patient wishes to die at home, as many but not all patients want to, then every effort is made to enable this to happen.

Hospices provide inpatient palliative care in units ranging from around 8 to 60 beds, the average being about 20. Larger units are staffed by one or more consultants in palliative medicine and full time junior staff while smaller units rely on sessional work by local general practitioners with experience in this area. Hospices admit patients for symptom control, terminal care, respite care (to give families a break of 1–2 weeks from caring for their relative) and intermediate care (supportive medical and nursing care following chemotherapy or radiotherapy). Hospices receive funding from a variety of sources, statutory and non-statutory.

Hospital palliative care teams are a relatively recent attempt to meet the needs of hospitalized patients. A typical team consists of one or two specialized nurses but in larger hospitals a multi-disciplinary team of consultants in palliative medicine and pain management, nurses, physiotherapists, psychologists and pharmacists might exist. The aim is to act in an advisory capacity to the referring team on symptom control and future management for the patient. Liaison with community teams and hospice units is an important aspect of the work.

Common symptom control problems	• Pain. • Nausea and vomiting. • Constipation. • Confusion. • Dyspnoea. • Dysphagia. • Intestinal obstruction.

In nearly all cases, these symptoms can be controlled to a tolerable level using the skills of a palliative care team.

Psychosocial care

Palliative care teams are able to offer advice and support for a number of psychosocial issues that often affect cancer patients and their relatives.

Feelings of sadness and somatic symptoms such as weight loss and anorexia are common to both advanced malignancy and depression. It is important to distinguish the two as depression is under-diagnosed in this population and does respond to a combination of drugs and psychological help.

Financial help is available in the form of allowances and grants from both the state and major charities to patients with advanced cancer. Palliative care teams can help the patient to claim these as well as facilitate the difficult process of making wills, funeral arrangements, etc.

Bereavement care

After a patient has died, most families grieve normally. This takes the form of:

• Accepting the reality of the loss.
• Working through the pain of grief.
• Adjusting to the new environment in which the deceased is missing.
• Emotionally relocating the deceased and moving on with life.

Although this process can take a year or two to complete, there are recognized indicators of a protracted or pathological bereavement. These include:

• The type of relationship with the deceased (e.g. ambivalent, highly dependent, one of abuse).

- Circumstances around the death (e.g. sudden death, perception of horrifying or mismanaged death, including poor symptom control).
- Characteristics of survivor (e.g. insecure, anxious, excessive anger).
- Social circumstances (e.g. lack of intimate others, unemployed, detached from cultural support systems).

Palliative care teams try to recognize these risk factors and adopt a proactive approach to bereavement care. These include liaison with the general practitioner and contacting the relative within a few weeks of the patients death to offer structured supportive visits to help the relative move through the grieving process.

Further reading

Doyle D, Hank G, Macdonald N. *Oxford Textbook of Palliative Medicine.* Oxford Medical Publications, 1997.

Related topics of interest

Breaking bad news (p. 26)
Nausea and vomiting (p. 167)
Pain control in cancer (p. 191)

PANCREATIC CANCER

Background

Incidence

Approximately 7000 cases of pancreatic cancer are diagnosed each year. It is the seventh most common cause of cancer death in the UK. The annual incidence is very close to the annual death rate because it is rarely curable. The incidence increases with age and varies in different geographical and ethnic groups.

Risk factors

Smoking is strongly associated with pancreatic cancer, with a relative risk of 2–3 compared with non-smokers, and is believed to be related to the pancreatic excretion of carcinogens such as the nitrosamines. Industrial exposure to these compounds is also associated with pancreatic cancer. Several other predisposing factors, such as diet, alcohol consumption and family history have been suggested, but few have been confirmed.

Aetiology

The aetiology is unknown. The molecular mechanisms of pathogenesis have not been defined, but there is a very high frequency of *ras* mutations in pancreatic cancer.

Histology

Ninety-five per cent of cancers arise from the exocrine portion of the pancreas, the majority in the proximal gland (head, neck and uncinate process) and only 20% in the body and 5–10% in the tail.

Ductal adenocarcinomas account for 85% of pancreatic cancers, the rest consisting of squamous carcinomas, sarcomas and giant cell cancers.

A small number of cancers arise from the endocrine glands as malignant islet cell tumours.

Clinical features

Presentation

The majority of patients present with advanced disease due to the highly malignant nature of pancreatic cancer. Local invasion often gives pain and leads to biliary or duodenal obstruction. Cachexia and anorexia are common and a higher incidence of depression has been reported compared to other GI malignancies. There is an increased incidence of venous thrombosis and migratory thrombophlebitis (Trousseau's sign).

Investigations

CT scanning is the radiological investigation of choice for diagnosis and to assess resectability. If resectability is in doubt CT angiography or MRI can be informative. ERCP can be helpful for the diagnosis of ductal lesions. If the tumour is deemed resectable, tissue for histological confirmation can be obtained at operation, otherwise pathological confirmation can be obtained by fine needle biopsy of the pancreas.

Serum levels of the tumour marker Ca19.9, are raised in 80% of pancreatic cancers. However, levels are increased with other upper GI cancers and with pancreatitis.

Staging

Staging of pancreatic cancer uses the TNM system:

T1   Confined to pancreas.
T2   Limited extension to duodenum, bile duct or peri-pancreatic tissues.
T3   Direct extension to stomach, spleen, colon or large vessel.

N0   No regional nodes.
N1   Regional nodes involved.
M0   No distant metastases.
M1   Metastases present.

Pancreatic cancer is frequently staged as follows:

Stage I: T1–2, N0, M0.
Stage II: T3,   N0, M0.
Stage III: T1–3, N1, M0.
Stage IV: T1–3, N0–1, M1.

Management

Surgery

Surgery is the only curative treatment for pancreatic cancer, but is only appropriate for a minority.

Surgery includes:

Intra-operative assessment. After exploration and direct visualization approximately only 20% are resectable.

Resection. If deemed possible, surgical resection involves a pancreatico-duodenectomy. More extensive surgery includes resection of the portal vein, superior mesenteric artery, coeliac axis and an extended nodal dissection. Whether a total pancreatic resection is always required is unresolved. Results of pancreatic surgery are best in specialist units which treat large numbers of patients.

If 'curable' resection is not possible, palliative bypass procedures to relieve biliary or gastric/duodenal obstruction may be performed.

Radiotherapy

Adjuvant radiotherapy post-operatively has not been proven to be of benefit. External beam radiotherapy can achieve useful palliation in patients with advanced disease.

Chemotherapy

Pancreatic cancer is resistant to chemotherapy. Combination chemotherapy with 5-FU and mitomycin-C has an response rate of approximately 25% but little impact on survival. Adjuvant chemotherapy post-operatively has not been demonstrated to have a useful role.

Prognostic factors

The most important prognostic factor is stage and hence resectability.

Screening

No screening procedure is available which can routinely detect early stage pancreatic cancer and therefore screening is not performed.

PARANEOPLASTIC SYNDROMES

Paraneoplastic syndromes are conditions occurring in the presence of a tumour that cannot be attributed to direct infiltration by the primary or metastatic disease.

Paraneoplastic syndromes may act as surrogate tumour markers. As such they may act as the presenting feature, be used to assess the response of the malignancy to treatment, or to suggest tumour relapse following treatment.

Incidence

Paraneoplastic syndromes occur in approximately 10% of patients. They occur more frequently with certain malignancies, for example small cell lung carcinoma, renal cell carcinomas.

Individual syndromes are classically associated with certain malignancies:

- Clubbing and squamous cell lung carcinoma.
- Lambert–Eaton syndrome and small cell lung carcinoma.
- Thrombophlebitis migrans and pancreatic carcinoma.

Aetiology

Two general mechanisms which may produce a paraneoplastic syndrome have been identified. These are:

- Excess production of hormones, growth factors or cytokines.
- Production of anti-tumour antibodies which cross-react with normal tissues.

The aetiology of many paraneoplastic syndromes remains obscure.

Clinical syndromes

Paraneoplastic syndromes include a diverse range of conditions which may affect any system. These include:

Endocrine

Secretion of hormones or their precursors by a tumour may lead to a diverse range of endocrine paraneoplastic syndromes.

1. Cushing's syndrome. Ectopic production of ACTH, most frequently seen with carcinomas of the lung, thymus and pancreas, may lead to Cushing's syndrome.

The paraneoplastic syndrome frequently occurs with rapid onset, marked weakness and metabolic disturbance (hypokalaemia, alkalosis and hyperglycaemia).

2. *SIADH.* The syndrome of inappropriate anti-diuretic hormone (ADH) is most frequently associated with small cell lung cancer where up to 40% of cases may have inappropriate ADH secretion.

3. *Others.* Other endocrine/metabolic disturbances seen include hypercalcaemia, hypoglycaemia and hyperglycaemia.

Neurological

Almost all neurological paraneoplastic syndromes are believed to be mediated by an autoimmune reaction to an antigen common to the tumour and the nervous system. Frequently, the neurological manifestations of the paraneoplastic syndrome present before the tumour is diagnosed.

1. *Lambert–Eaton myasthenic syndrome.* This is characterised by weakness and fatiguability principally affecting proximal muscles. Autonomic dysfunction may also occur. Deep tendon reflexes are lost but may return after attempts to contract the muscle. The syndrome is caused by antibodies directed against voltage-gated calcium channels. More than 50% are associated with small cell lung cancer. Other causes include thymoma and lymphoma.

2. *Sub-acute cerebellar degeneration.* This may lead to incapacitating symptoms. Small cell lung, breast and ovary cancer and Hodgkin's disease are the most frequent neoplastic associations. Specific autoantibodies have been identified

3. *Others.* Other neurological paraneoplastic syndromes include peripheral neuropathies and Guillain–Barre syndrome.

Muscle/joint

1. *HPOA.* Hypertrophic pulmonary osteoarthropathy (HPOA) is associated with malignant disease in more

than 90% of cases (most frequently with bronchal carcinoma). In addition to digital clubbing, periosteal new bone formation occurs, leading to pain over the distal ends of the ulnar/radius and tibia/fibula and a characteristic X-ray appearance.

2. *Dermatomyositis/polymyositis.* These idiopathic inflammatory myopathies are characterized by immune-mediated muscle inflammation, leading to weakness. Polymyositis presents as proximal muscle weakness; dermatomyositis has additional characteristic dermatological findings. Dermatomyositis and polymyositis are associated with malignancy in approximately 1 in 4 patients. A wide variety of malignancies have been associated, including ovarian and stomach.

3. *Others.* Other rheumatic paraneoplastic syndromes include polyarthritis.

Haematological

Paraneoplastic syndromes may affect any component of the haematological system.

1. *Thrombosis.* The association of thrombosis with malignancy is well described (Trousseau's syndrome). Recurrent idiopathic deep venous thrombosis (DVT) has been demonstrated to be associated with an overt malignancy in almost one in six patients.

2. *Anaemia.* The most common anaemia of cancer is characteriszed by a normochromic normocytic anaemia with normal or raised ferritin levels and a low reticulocyte count. Low levels of endogenous erythropoietin are believed to be pathogenic. Haemolytic anaemia due to autoimmune destruction of red cells is seen in lymphoproliferative disorders.

3. *Others.* Polycythaemia, granulocytosis, neutropenia and platelet disorders are also recognized paraneoplastic syndromes.

Dermatological

1. *Acanthosis nigricans.* This describes pruritic, pigmented hyperkeratotic plaques classically affecting

the axillae. More than half of the paraneoplastic cases are associated with stomach cancer.

2. Others. Pruritus, vitiligo, erythema multiforme, hyperkeratosis of the palms and soles and erythroderma are also recognized paraneoplastic syndromes.

Miscellaneous

1. Clubbing. Clubbing is most frequently associated with bronchial carcinomas (particularly squamous cell carcinoma), renal carcinoma, naso-pharyngeal carcinoma and Hodgkin's disease. It is also associated with non-malignant conditions such as pulmonary fibrosis, pulmonary sepsis, inflammatory bowel disease, cyanotic heart disease and HIV infection. The cause remains unknown although there are several theories including the release of growth factors.

2. Cachexia. Cancer-associated cachexia, characterized by anorexia, weight loss and weakness, is probably the most frequent paraneoplastic syndrome, (occuring in up to 80% of patients with upper GI malignancies). It is probably mediated by a number of factors including cytokines such as TNF-α and IL-1.

3. Fever. Production of cytokines such as TNF-α and IL-1 may also lead to a paraneoplastic fever. This is particularly frequent in leukaemias and lymphomas but is also seen with solid tumours.

Further reading

Nathanson L, Hall T. Paraneoplastic syndromes. *Seminars in Oncology,* Vol. 24, no. 3.

Related topic of interest

Hypercalcaemia (p. 116)
Lung cancer (p. 136)

POLYMERASE CHAIN REACTION

Definition

The polymerase chain reaction (PCR) is a molecular biology technique capable of generating multiple copies of a given sequence of DNA. Using PCR, over a million copies of such DNA sequences can be obtained from as little as a single cell. This provides sufficient quantities of DNA for diagnostic, research and forensic applications.

Biology

PCR is dependent on the ability of the enzyme DNA polymerase to synthesize the complementary strand of DNA from a single-stranded DNA template (*Figure 1*). DNA polymerase can only add nucleotides to a pre-existing sequence. In the PCR reaction these sequences are provided by 'primers', oligonucleotides approximately 20 base pairs long with the specific DNA sequence required to bind to the target template DNA. Specific primers are required for a particular PCR reaction and therefore their design requires prior knowledge of the target DNA sequence.

The 'ingredients' of a PCR reaction are:

- Target template DNA (as little as a single copy).
- Primers (commercially synthesized).
- DNA polymerase.
- Free nucleotides (guanine, adenosine, cytosine, thymidine).
- Reaction buffer to create the correct reaction environment (e.g. Mg^{2+} concentration).

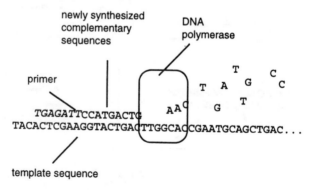

Figure 1. DNA polymerase.

The DNA polymerase most commonly used for PCR is from the bacterium *Thermophilus aquaticus (Taq)* because the enzyme from this organism is stable at the high temperatures used.

PCR (*Figure 2*) is carried out in micro test-tubes or microwell plates in volumes of 25–100 μl. The following steps are performed in a thermocycler, a machine capable of accurately regulating the reaction temperature.

1. Denaturation. The sample is heated approximately 95°C for 1 min to separate the strands.

2. Annealing. The primers are bound to the single-stranded DNA at each end of the target sequence (1 min at approximately 60°C).

3. Extension. The complementary stand is extended by DNA polymerase at approximately 72°C for 1 min.

This cycle is then repeated. After one cycle there are two copies, after two cycles there are four copies and after 30 cycles there are 2^{30} (1×10^8) copies.

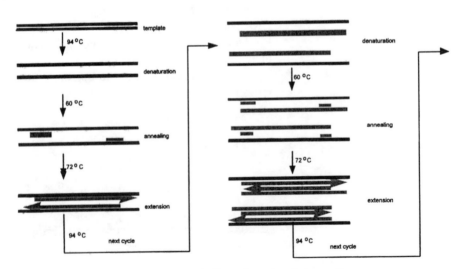

Figure 2. The polymerase chain reaction.

Uses

PCR is particularly useful when trying to detect very small quantities of DNA, either when very little tissue is available for analysis or when very small numbers of abnormal cells are present.

Diagnostic

1. *Diagnostic aids.*

- Detection of translocations associated with particular conditions [e.g. the *bcr-abl* translocation (the Philadelphia chromosome) in chronic myeloid leukaemia].
- Detection of point mutations associated with diseases (e.g. inherited gene disorders such as sickle cell disease and cystic fibrosis).
- Detection of DNA sequences of infectious agents (e.g. Mycobacterium, Mycoplasma, HIV).

2. *Detection of sub-clinical malignant disease.*

- To detect the presence of translocations only found in malignant cells (e.g. the *bcr-abl* translocation).
- To detect the presence of lymphomas by detecting the particular sequences of the variable region of antibody genes in malignant clones.
- To detect the expression of tissue-specific genes (e.g. the melanocyte-specific gene tyrosinase) in tissues not normally expressing these genes (e.g. the detection of circulating melanoma cells by the detection of tyrosinase gene expression in blood).

Research

- Isolation of genes to detect mutations or other differences in sequence between normal and abnormal cells to characterize the genetic defects in acquired and inherited conditions.
- Isolation of novel genes that are similar in sequence to previously identified genes.
- Isolation of genes for genetic engineering.

Forensic

- To amplify DNA for 'DNA fingerprinting'.
- To compare DNA samples at the scene of the crime with those of a suspect.
- To amplify DNA samples from two subjects to establish parentage.

The use of PCR is now being applied to virtually all branches of medicine and science from archaeology to pre-natal diagnosis.

Further reading

Markham AF. The polymerase chain reaction: a tool for molecular medicine. *British Medical Journal,* 1993; **306:** 441–6.
Newton CR, Graham A. *PCR,* 2nd Edn. Oxford: BIOS Scientific Publishers, 1997.

PRIMARY UNKNOWN (CANCER OF UNKNOWN ORIGIN)

In up to 10% of patients with histologically proven malignancy, the site of the primary tumour remains unknown following standard investigations. Even following thorough investigation some 3% of tumours have unknown primaries.

The importance of further investigations depends on each clinical situation. Factors needing consideration include age and fitness of the patient, the possible sites of the primary cancer, the prognosis and potential for therapy for the possible primary tumours, and the invasiveness and availability of investigations.

Predicting the site of primary cancer

Clinical features of the patient will provide clues to the possible sites and guide further investigations. Other useful indicators to predict the primary site include the following.

Site of metastases	Common primaries
Liver	colon, lung, breast
Lung	breast, lung, kidney
Brain	lung, breast, melanoma
Bone	breast, bronchus, kidney, prostate, thyroid
Peritoneal	ovary, GI tract (esp. stomach), pancreas
Lymph nodes	
High cervical	head and neck, thyroid, lung
Lower cervical/supra-clavicular	head and neck, lung, breast, GI tract
Axillary	breast, lung, melanoma
Inguinal	ovary, prostate, ano-rectal, vulva
Histology	Histology may help to identify a tissue type of origin. The majority of carcinomas of unknown primary are adenocarcinomas or undifferentiated tumours, rarely squamous cell carcinoma, melanoma, sarcoma and neuroendocrine tumours. The most likely primary sites for particular types of histology are:

- Adenocarcinoma: GI tract (including pancreas), breast, ovary and lung.
- Squamous: lung, head and neck.

Further investigations

These are targetted to detect treatable options, that is primaries which indicate a likely benefit from local systemic therapy. It is important to avoid unpleasant, invasive investigations which are unlikely to benefit the patient even if an additional piece of diagnostic information is forthcoming.

Standard investigations   All patients should have:

- Full clinical assessment and examinations.
- Panel of tumour markers.
- Chest X-ray.
- Pathology review.

Additional investigations   Most patients should have:

- Abdominal and thoracic non-invasive imaging (CT, UV or MRI).
- Immunophenotyping of the histological specimens can provide more accurate predictions of the primary site.

Specific investigations   Some patients, where clinical indications suggest a possible treatable diagnosis should have:

- Barium studies.
- Endoscopies.
- Bone marrow biopsy.
- Mammograms.

Management

If no conclusive decision as to the primary can be made, treatment will depend on several factors:

- Age and fitness of the patient.
- Likely primary sites.
- Responsiveness of potential primaries to treatment.

Essentially, treatment is aimed at treatable tumours that may be the primary tumour. For example, in a young male with a midline tumour of differentiated cancer, even without raised germ cell markers (i.e. a possible germ cell origin), it may be reasonable to try BEP chemotherapy. Treatable tumours against which treatment is aimed are mainly germ cell tumours, breast cancer and ovarian cancer. Chemotherapeutic regimens that include an anthracyline and a platinum agent will cover these tumours and can be combined with 5-FU which has activity in many GI tumours. In patients too unwell to receive chemotherapy, hormonal treatment with tamoxifen may be considered if breast cancer is a possibility. Radiotherapy can be given for palliation of symptoms, for example bone pain.

Prognostic factors

Overall, the prognosis for patients with cancer of unknown origin is poor, with a median survival of approximately 3–4 months. Five year survival is less than 10%. Poor prognostic features include male sex, increasing number of organ sites, adenocarcinoma histology and hepatic involvement.

Further reading

Lindeman GJ, Tattersall M. In: Peckham M, Priedo HM, Veronesi U, eds. *Oxford Textbook of Oncology.* Oxford University Press, 1995; 2155–65.

Related topics of interest

Chemotherapy – (a) general principles (p. 48)
Metastases (p. 147)
Tumour markers (p. 263)

PROSTATE CANCER

Background

Incidence

Prostate cancer is the third most common cancer in males with more than 10 000 new cases diagnosed in the UK each year. It is predominantly a disease of older men, with more than 50% occuring over the age of 75.

Aetiology

There are no clear aetiologicals agents, although radiation exposure, diet and anabolic steroids have all been implicated. These may alter the level of the male hormone testosterone which controls the growth, and function of the prostate. Mutations of *BRCA II* and the *pTEN* genes are associated with an increased risk but familial prostate cancer is rare.

Histology

Over 95% of tumours are adenocarcinomas developing in glandular tissue in the posterior or peripheral part of the prostate gland. Benign prostatic hyperplasia more commonly arises in the centre of the gland. Histological grade and architecture, defined by the Gleason grade, affects prognosis. Within any tumour, different foci may vary in their degree of differentiation from indolent to aggressive.

Clinical features

Presentation

Prostatic cancer is frequently asymptomatic and diagnosed by routine rectal examination. Patients may present with symptoms of prostatism, including poor stream, nocturia, dribbling and increased frequency. Some patients present with metastatic symptoms, commonly bone pain.

Examination

Characteristically on rectal examination an enlarged, hard, craggy gland is felt, with obliteration of the median sulcus.

Investigation

Histological diagnosis is mandatory with a transrectal biopsy ideally performed under ultrasound guidance with multiple sampling of different areas being performed. This also allows the size of the gland to be assessed. Several tumour markers can be measured but the serum prostate-specific antigen (PSA) is the most commonly used, with more overall sensitivity and specificity than other markers. Radionuclide bone scans may be useful to detect bone metastases. MRI more clearly defines the extent of extracapsular spread.

Staging

The TNM staging system:

T0   No palpable tumour.
T1   Intracapsular tumour surrounded by normal prostatic tissue.
T2   Tumour confined to the gland but with deformity and minimal capsule invasion.
T3   Tumour extends locally beyond the capsule (including invasion of the seminal vesicles).
T4   Tumour fixed or involving local structures.

N0   No regional lymph node involvement.
N1   Regional lymph node involvement (single).
N2   Regional lymph node involvement (multiple).
N3   More widespread nodal involvement.

M0   No known metastases.
M1   Distant metastases (usually bone).

Several grading systems for prostate cancer exist. The Gleason system scores tumours (from 2 to 10) on the basis of histological patterns in the two most predominant areas of the tumour.

Management

Prostatic cancer is relatively indolent and in some cases occurs in elderly patients who may die from concomitant medical problems. Locally advanced disease may be treated with surgery, radiotherapy and/or systemic therapy. The choice of treatment modality is guided by factors including age of patient, performance status, presence of other medical conditions and to some degree the preference of individual clinicians.

Observation

In patients with asymptomatic disease, confined to the prostate, observation rather than active treatment may be appropriate. The optimum management of patients with an elevated PSA but no clinical evidence of prostate cancer is unknown.

Surgery	In patients with localized disease (T2 disease or less) radical prostatectomy with curative intent can be performed by perineal or retroperineal routes. There are, however, significant side effects of impotence and incontinence. Surgery even in a selected population of fitter patients can be associated with a 1–2% mortality.

In patients with localized disease (T2 disease or less) radical prostatectomy with curative intent can be performed by perineal or retroperineal routes. There are, however, significant side effects of impotence and incontinence. Surgery even in a selected population of fitter patients can be associated with a 1–2% mortality.

Palliative surgical techniques such as trans-urethral resections may be used to relieve prostatic symptoms or urinary obstruction

Radiotherapy

Radical radiotherapy may be used as an alternative to surgery in T1 and T2 tumours. It is also more appropriate for the control of more advanced local disease. Adjuvant radiotherapy may also be given following radical surgery. Definitive radiotherapy should be delayed until at least 6 weeks following transurethral resection to prevent stricture formation. Radiotherapy may be performed by external beam irradiation, by the interstitial implantation of radioisotopes (brachytherapy) or by a combination of these.

Palliative radiotherapy is used to both palliate the primary tumour and to treat metastatic complications.

Chemotherapy

Cytotoxic drugs have been found to give disappointing results and are not routinely used. Hormone-resistant metastatic disease may be treated with combination chemotherapy.

Hormonal therapy

Hormonal treatments are used in advanced disease. Inhibition of the growth-stimulatory effect of endogenous androgens may effectively treat prostatic cancer with a response rate of approximately 80%. Hormonal manipulation can also be used in a neoadjuvant manner to 'downstage' a tumour prior to surgery.

A variety of hormonal options are available:

1. LHRH agonists. Lutenizing-hormone releasing hormone (LHRH) interferes with the normal release of gonadotrophins from the pituatary, This reduces the level of circulating testosterone to those following castration. Agents include goserelin and buserelin. Side effects include impotence, loss of libido and tumour flare. Tumour flare occurs on initiation of treatment (prior to the down regulation of gonadotrophin and may be treated by short-term concomitant anti-androgen therapy.

2. Oestrogen therapy. Oestrogens inhibit LHRH production from the hypothalmus. They are rarely used because of their side effects: impotence, loss of libido; gynaecomastia; myocardial infarction; cerebro-vascular accidents (CVAs); and pulmonary emboli. LHRH agonists have largely replaced the use of oestrogens.

3. Anti-androgens. These compounds compete with androgens for sites on the androgen receptor. They include flutamide, cyproterone acetate, megestrol acetate and medroxyprogesterone acetate.

4. Bilateral orchidectomy. Although previously the standard option, orchidectomy is less commonly performed today.

Prognostic factors

Survival is related to the extent of the tumour. The median survival for patients with locally advanced tumours is 4.5 years. Following radical surgery or radiotherapy, the 10 year survival for localized disease reaches 80–90%. Patients with metastatic disease have a median survival of 2.5 years. High levels of serum PSA and serum acid phosphatase are associated with a poorer prognosis.

Screening

Digital rectal examination and serum PSA are able to detect early stage prostate cancer. The role of screening in the general population is unclear and it is not routinely performed in the UK. The value of screening is currently being assessed.

Current issues

The value of screening is being investigated (see above). The relevance of raised tumour markers and borderline histological findings is being assessed along with the role of the role of surgery or surveillance in such cases.

Molecular genetics   The identification of the genes responsible for the development and the progression of prostatic cancer is being investigated. This includes the detection of the genes responsible for familial cases. The *pTEN* gene, which has an association with prostate cancer, has recently been cloned.

Further reading

Dawson C, Whitfield H. ABC of oncology: oncological malignancy – prostate cancer. *British Medical Journal,* 1996; **312:** 1032–4.
Frydenberg M, Stricker PD, Kaye KW. Prostate cancer diagnosis and management. *Lancet,* 1997; **349:** 1681–7.

Related topic of interest

Biological therapy (p. 7)

QUALITY OF LIFE

An assessment of quality of life (QL) is used to measure well-being and to monitor the outcome of treatment. Patients with cancer may suffer more emotional distress and morbidity than patients with chronic life-threatening illnesses such as ischaemic heart disease. In addition, many cancer treatments given with palliative intent are associated with significant toxicity. The assessment of QL is therefore an important part of modern cancer management and is becoming an integral part of assessing response to treatment.

Definition

Quality of life has been defined as:

- The subjective evaluation of life as a whole.
- Patients' appraisal of and satisfaction with their current level of functioning compared with what they perceive to be possible or ideal.
- Physical, mental and social well-being, not merely the absence of disease or infirmity (WHO).

Measurement

The accurate assessment of QL requires an assessment of many areas of the individual's life:

1. Physical functioning. This includes performance of self-care activities, functional status, mobility, physical activities, and 'role activities' such as work or household responsibilities.

2. Disease- and treatment-related symptoms. This includes specific symptoms from the disease such as pain, shortness of breath or side effects of drug therapy such as nausea, vomiting, hair loss.

3. Psychological functioning. Meaning emotional distress, anxiety, depression that may be secondary to the disease.

4. Social functioning. For example family interactions, time with friends, recreation activities.

5. Others. Additional considerations in the evaluation of QL may include:

- Spiritual or existential concerns.

- Cognitive function.
- Sexual functioning and body image.
- Satisfaction with health care.

QL instruments

During the past decade there has been a rapid expansion of psychometric assays (instruments) used to assess QL in patients with cancer. These include:

1. Generic. This is not specifically designed for cancer patients. This catagory includes Medical Outcome Study (MOS), SF-36 (short form of MOS), Nottingham Health Profile (NHP), Sickness Impact Profile (SIP).

2. Cancer specific. This includes, for example EORTC Core QL Questionnaire, Rotterdam Symptom Checklist (RSCL), FACT scale (functional assessment of cancer therapy).

3. Cancer site specific. Includes, for example Breast Cancer Chemotherapy Questionnaire, EORTC Lung Cancer Module.

4. QL domain specific instruments. These include:

- Psychiatric diagnostic tools: Hospital Anxiety and Depression (HAD) Scale, General Health Questionnaire.
- General physical functioning: Karnofsky performance status, WHO performance status.
- General symptomatology: Memorial Symptom Assessment Scale (MSAS).
- Nausea and vomiting: Morrow assessment of nausea and emesis (MANE), Rhodes index of nausea and vomiting (INV).
- Pain: McGill pain questionnaire (MPQ), Memorial pain assessment card (MPAC).

Most instruments have been designed for self-administration and are relatively short, allowing their use in clinical trials. Some of the QL instruments (indexes) generate a single QL score, others (profiles) generate several scores on different QL domains.

Clinical applications of QL measurement

Clinical trials

An assessment of QL in clinical trials is increasingly being used as an outcome measure, usually in addition to traditional measures, such as tumour response and survival.

Some important observations about QL have been made:

- More aggressive anti-cancer treatment can be associated with an improved QL (e.g. continuous vs. intermittent chemotherapy for breast cancer).
- A more effective therapy is usually associated with better QL, even if it is more intensive and associated with toxic effects.
- Patients may report an improved QL despite showing no objective response. This could be related to minimal shrinkage of the tumour, giving relief to symptoms, to increased medical attention, or to provision of hope.
- Descriptive studies have confirmed the clinical feeling that symptoms of cancer are associated with quantifiable disruptions in QL.
- Pre-treatment QL status may predict survival in metastatic breast cancer, lung cancer and melanoma.

Health economics

QL measurements provide another parameter for assessing treatment options for health planning. These often use parameters combining quality and quantity of life, for example quality-adjusted life years (QALY) of survival or quality of time without symptoms or treatment side effects (Q-TWIST)

Psychosocial oncology

QL instruments and psychiatric diagnostic tools can be used for the identification of emotional distress and key problem areas that require intervention. The HAD scale and Rotterdam checklist have been shown to be useful instruments for screening for psychiatric morbidity (depression and anxiety). Their detection rate has been demonstrated as superior to that of doctors and nurses involved in cancer care.

Further reading

De Haes JCKM, Zittoun RA. Quality of Life. In: *Oxford Textbook of Oncology*, Oxford University Press, 1994; 2400–8.

Ganz PA. Quality of life and the patient with cancer. *Cancer*, 1994; **74:** 1445–52.

Osoba D. Lessons learned from measuring health-related quality of life in oncology. *Journal of Clinical Oncology*, 1995; **12:** 608–16.

RADIOBIOLOGY

Radiobiology is the study of the effects of ionizing radiation on living things and explains some of the rationale behind current radiotherapy practices.

Cellular response   Radiotherapy affects both normal and tumour cells through the induction of DNA damage. Ionizing radiation produces fast charged particles by interaction with the atoms of the material, the exact mode depending on the energy of the incident beam. These particles directly or indirectly (via production of free radicals) damage DNA. If not repaired, this may lead to cell death by apoptosis.

Cell cycle   Cells are generally most radiosensitive in the M and G2 phases of the cell cycle and most resistant in the S phase. The delivery of a single dose of radiotherapy to a population of cells evenly distributed around the cell cycle causes disproportionate killing of those cells in the radiosensitive phases of the cycle. Delivery of a second dose will increase cell killing as some cells previously radioresistant will have entered radiosensitive phases of the cell cycle. Such re-assortment confers theoretical advantages to fractionated regimes.

Normal tissue reaction

Optimal radiotherapy delivery produces maximum tumour cell kill but spares normal tissues. The therapeutic window is a compromise between the toxicity to tumour cells and that to normal tissue. The toxicity produced can be divided into early and late effects.

Early effects   These occur at or around the time of treatment and are self-limiting. The reactions are seen in rapidly proliferating tissues where the effects of radiotherapy are expressed early. Examples include radiation-induced colitis and mucositis. Prolongation of the treatment schedule will reduce early effects.

Late effects   These may develop many years after radiotherapy. Vulnerable tissues are very slowly dividing and may not express their radiation-induced damage for many years. The resultant tissue damage is permanent and often impairs function. It therefore heavily influences treatment practices. Examples include myelitis and radiation-induced cataracts.

Radiation carcinogenesis

- Probability increases with dose and there may be no threshold.
- Severity is independent of dose.
- The latency between exposure and malignancy varies, e.g. 5–7 years for leukaemia and up to 50 years for solid tumours.
- Regardless of the age of exposure, radiation-induced cancers normally appear at the same age as one would expect to see spontaneous tumours.

Fractionation

Radiotherapy is delivered in a single large dose or more commonly split into smaller equal doses or fractions over a more prolonged period. Both the delivery of multiple fractions and the consequent prolongation in overall treatment time confer advantages to normal tissues. These benefits are explained by the following effects:

Effects

- Repair in normal tissues of sub-lethal DNA damage between the fractions. This is maximal in those tissues exhibiting late effects.
- Repopulation of the normal tissues occurs due to cellular proliferation taking place during the protracted treatment times. Rapidly dividing tissues will benefit most and early effects are therefore reduced. Excessive prolongation may allow tumour proliferation and subsequent reduction in tumour control, however.
- Re-assortment of the tumour cells into the more radiosensitive areas of the cell cycle.
- Re-oxygenation of tumour cells during fractionation. Hypoxic cells are relatively radioresistant. The tumour becomes better perfused as the tumour mass reduces.

Hyperfractionation

Normal radiotherapy practice is to deliver one fraction per day. However, there are some advantages to giving smaller fractions twice or even three times per day. Overall treatment time is identical to conventional dosing. The effect is to reduce late effects and allow larger doses to be used to improve tumour control.

	Trials in head and neck cancers have reported 15% improved local control.
Accelerated treatment	Delivering two conventionally sized fractions per day allows treatment time to be halved. The total dose and number of fractions are identical to standard treatments. The shorter overall treatment time reduces repopulation in rapidly proliferating tissues. There will be improved control in fast-dividing tumours at the expense of exaggerated early effects.

Further reading

Hall EJ. *Radiobiology for the Radiologist,* 4th edn. Philadelphia: JB Lippincott Co., 1994.

Related topics of interest

Cell cycle (p. 40)
Radiotherapy – principles (p. 224)

RADIOTHERAPY – PRINCIPLES

Radiotherapy is given to 25–35% of cancer patients in the UK each year. It is used with curative intent in two thirds of these patients, either used alone or in conjunction with other treatment modalities. Many other patients will receive palliative radiotherapy to help to relieve the symptoms associated with metastatic disease.

Indications

Radical

Radiotherapy is given over a protracted period with curative intent. Examples include:

- Head and neck cancers.
- Cervical cancer.
- Bladder cancer.
- Inoperable early lung cancer.
- Lymphomas.
- Inoperable early oesophageal cancer.

Adjuvant

Treatment is given after 'complete' surgical resection to improve local disease control. This is now the accepted practice following wide local excision in breast cancer and in rectal cancer (Dukes' C).

Neoadjuvant

Radiotherapy may be used pre-operatively in the hope of improving local disease control, for example in rectal cancer, and may improve survival.

Post-operative

This is used when there is residual disease. Often the site of such disease is marked at the original operation by metal clips to aid localization.

Palliative

Radiotherapy can be used to enhance the quality of life in patients with recurrent or metastatic disease. Some examples of its use are:

- Painful bone metastases.
- Compression of vital structures, e.g. spinal cord compression, oesophageal or bronchial obstruction.
- Brain metastases.

Treatment delivery

This can be given as:

External beam X-rays, γ-rays, or electrons emitted from an external source incident on the skin and deposit energy either superficially or more deeply, depending on the characteristics of the beam.

Brachytherapy Radioactive sources are placed within body cavities or into tumours to produce a high dose of radiation to the local vicinity only, for example to treat cervical carcinoma.

Radionuclides Certain radioisotopes are avidly taken up by particular tumour cells and cell death results from the emitted radiation, for example the treatment of thyroid cancer with iodine-131.

X-ray production

Kilovoltage X-rays These are produced when electrons emitted from a heated metal filament are accelerated into a high-atomic-weight metal target by applying a potential difference across them.

Megavoltage X-rays/electrons These are both produced by the same machine, a linear accelerator. The electrons from a heated filament are directed along a wave-guide which accelerates them to very high speeds within a relatively short distance. These then impinge upon a target to produce high-energy X-rays. Alternatively, the target is simply removed from the incident beam to produce electrons.

Gamma rays These are identical to X-rays but are produced by unstable nuclei. Cobalt-60 produces γ-rays of 1.2 MeV energy. This may be used for external beam delivery or brachytherapy.

External beam radiation

Several different types of radiation are used:

Superficial This describes photon energies up to 150 kV. The dose to the skin is high but falls off rapidly with depth. It is ideal for superficial skin cancers.

Orthovoltage	Photon energies up to 300 kV provide slightly better penetration than superficial energies, and are used in the treatment of rib metastases, for example.
Megavoltage	These energies have far superior penetration and are necessary to deliver uniform doses to deep structures. Additionally, there is no preferential bone absorption and the maximum dose is delivered just below the surface. This 'skin sparing' effect reduces the skin reaction often seen during treatment. Higher energy beams produce superior dose penetration.
Electrons	These are directly ionizing and have a finite range in tissues. The skin and adjacent tissues receive a relatively uniform dose which falls off abruptly, at depth. This well-defined peak of energy is useful if deep-lying critical structures are to be avoided. The depth–dose characteristics depend on the energy of the beam.
Treatment delivery	External-beam radiotherapy aims to deliver a homogeneous tumourcidal dose of radiation to a pre-defined tumour volume and to spare normal tissues as much as possible. Localization of the tumour volume requires clinical examination, radiological investigations and a knowledge of the likely routes of spread. Once this has been defined the following steps are pursued:

- Define the target volume. This includes the tumour volume plus a margin of normal tissue. This region is likely to contain microscopic disease.
- Relate the target volume to fixed markers on the skin surface.

The above two steps can be quickly acheived by a simulator. This is an isocentrically mounted diagnostic X-ray machine connected to an image intensifier. The set-up is the same as on a treatment machine and therefore provides a beam's eye view of the treatment volume. Guide wires define this and by convention are equivalent to the 50% isodose line. The field size is projected onto the patients skin and the centre tattooed.

- Use the various physical properties of different types of radiation (superficial, megavoltage or electrons) to produce an homogeneous dose covering the target volume and sparing vital structures such as the spinal cord.

- A dose is then prescribed that will be tumourcidal but limits damage to the surrounding tissues.
- Treatment delivery is by trained therapeutic radiographers.
- During the treatment the dose and field arrangements are checked by computer verification systems.

Brachytherapy

Radioactive sources are placed adjacent to or within a tumour. High doses are delivered to the immediate vicinity, but dose levels decline rapidly with increasing distance from the sources according to the inverse square law.

Accurate placement is essential. Systems have been developed which describe the necessary distribution and activity of the sources needed to achieve a particular dose at a defined reference point. Caesium-137 and iridium-192 are the commonest sources used. Often empty applicators are positioned in theatre and the patient is then transferred to a shielded room where radioactive sources are introduced into the applicators via remote control. This avoids any exposure of the staff to radiation.

Radionuclides

Certain radioisotopes are avidly taken up by particular tumour cells often producing cell death. Examples include iodine-131 used in the treatment of thyroid cancer, strontium-89 used in osteoblastic bone metastases and MIBG (metaiodobenzyl-guanidine) used for neuroblastomas.

Current issues

CHART Continuous hyperfractionated accelerated radiotherapy. Several fractions are given each day over a much shorter time period. This attempts to overcome proliferation of rapidly growing tumour cells during treatment.

PET scanning The use of positron emission tomography (PET) scanning in an attempt to improve localization of tumours prior to radiation planning.

Further reading

Dobbs J, Barrett A, Ash D. *Practical Radiotherapy Planning.* Edward Arnold Publisher, 1992.

Related topics of interest

Cell cycle (p. 40)
Chemotherapy – (a) general principles (p. 48)
Radiobiology (p. 221)

RENAL CANCER

Background

Incidence

Renal cancers account for 2% of all cancers in the UK, with approximately 5000 new cases each year. Renal cancers are three times more common in men than women and the peak incidence is in the sixth and seventh decades.

Aetiology

Renal cell carcinoma (RCC) is associated with smoking, cystic disease of the kidney and long-term dialysis. Recent evidence suggests that an oncogene located on the short arm of chromosome 3 may be implicated. Of the renal cell carcinomas, 1% are familial, the commonest associated syndrome being the Von Hippel-Lindau syndrome.

Histology

Adenocarcinomas (also known as hypernephroma, clear-cell carcinoma or Grawitz tumours) constitute 85% of adult renal cancers. They are believed to arise from the proximal renal tubular epithelium. Transitional cell carcinomas, squamous carcinomas and lymphomas can also arise in the kidney. Tumours of the renal pelvis are uncommon and account for about 10%. Wilm's tumours occur principally in children. RCC spreads by local, lymphatic and haematogenous spread.

Clinical features

Presentation

The classical features are haematuria (60%), loin pain (45%) and a palpable mass (35%) although only 5% have the classical triad. Many renal carcinomas present late with diverse symptoms. 25% have locally advanced tumours and 30% have metastatic disease at presentation. Other features at presentation include those due to metastases which most commonly occur in the lungs and bones. Paraneoplastic syndromes are well recognized and include pyrexias of unknown origin, hypertension, polycythaemia and hypercalcaemia.

| Investigations | A histological diagnosis is mandatory, with biopsy of the primary or a metastatic site. Urinalysis and cytological examination of the urine may also demonstrate malignancy. Staging investigations include CXR, CT of abdomen, pelvis and chest and a bone scan. If a nephrectomy is considered it is important to assess the renal function of the contralateral kidney. |

Staging

There are several staging systems presently used. The TNM classification is:

TX	Primary tumour can not be assessed.
TO	No evidence of primary tumour.
T1	Tumour less than 2.5 cm limited to the kidney.
T2	Tumour more 2.5 cm limited to the kidney.
T3	Perinephric or renal vein involvement.
T4	Invasion of neighbouring structures (diaphragm and abdominal wall).

N0	No nodal involvement.
N1	Metastases in a single lymph node less than 2 cm.
N2	Metastases in a single lymph node greater than 2 cm and less than 5 cm.
N3	Metastases in a lymph node greater than 5 cm.

| M0 | No known distant metastases. |
| M1 | Distant metastases. |

The most commonly used staging system is the Robson staging.

Stage 1:	Confined to kidney.
Stage 2:	Perirenal fat involvement, but confined to Gerota's fascia.
Stage 3A:	Gross renal vein/inferior vena cava involvement.
Stage 3B:	Lymphatic involvement.
Stage 3C:	Vascular and lymphatic involvement.
Stage 4A:	Adjacent organs other than adrenal involvement.
Stage 4B:	Distant metastases.

Management

Surgery

Resection of a localized tumour is the most effective treatment and is possible for approximately 70% of patients at presentation. Localized disease (stages 1–3) is curable with a radical nephrectomy which includes removal of the kidney and adrenal gland. Surgery, with more radical local resection may be appropriate in more advanced local disease (e.g. local extension into adjacent structures), as this can improve survival and local control. For smaller tumours (some stage 1) simple resection or partial nephrectomy may be appropriate.

Some patients with small volume metastases and good performance status should be considered for a nephrectomy as this may improve local control and there are data to suggest that patients with minimal bulk disease respond better to biological therapies.

In patients who are unfit for surgery and symptomatic from their RCC the supplying artery can be embolized: this procedure will control localized symptoms such as pain and bleeding.

Radiotherapy

Renal cell carcinoma is a radioresistant tumour. This is thought to be partly due to the poor vascularization of the tumour and the slow growth rate. Therefore radiotherapy is not routinely used either as an adjuvant post-operatively or as first line treatment. However, radiotherapy can be used effectively to control the symptoms from metastatic sites, in particular bone and brain.

Chemotherapy

Renal cell carcinoma is also very chemoresistant and most response rates to single or combination therapy are disappointing. The best single agent activity is with vinblastine, although only occasional responses are seen.

Hormonal therapy

The overall response to progestogens and androgens is less than 5%. Medroxy progesterone acetate is a widely used hormonal agent which is tolerated well with minimal side effects. It has the advantage of making the patients feel well initially whilst on the treatment.

Biological therapy

Biological therapies continue to be evaluated in RCC due to the disappointing response rates of conventional therapies and to the anecdodal evidence that an immune response can be mounted against RCC. In particular, some long-lasting remissions have been seen with biological agents.

Single-agent IFN has a response rate in metastatic renal cancer of approximately 15% and has recently been shown to increase the survival of patients significantly. The doses examined range from very low dose (which appears to have no effect) to intermediate doses (which have some some effect with tolerable toxicity). The effect is most likely a combination of a direct anti-proliferative effect and an enhancement of host anti-tumour responses. There is promise with IFN used in combination with other agents [e.g. interleukin-2 (IL-2) and 5-FU], which has response rates up to 30–40% in selected patients. The use of interferon alone in post-operative adjuvant therapy appears to have little effect.

IL-2 as a single agent has response rates in metastatic RCC of between 10 and 15%. The inital studies involved the use of very high dose bolus IL-2 associated with severe toxicity. Intermediate dose IL-2 appears to have similar efficacy but with less toxicity. Its use is still being evaluated in clinical trials, alone and in combination.

Prognostic factors

As in most tumour types, the prognosis depends on stage, histological grade and completeness of surgery. Patients with advanced renal cell carcinoma have a poor prognosis with a median survival (after diagnosis of metastases) of approximately 8 months. Survival is related to stage, with a 5 year survival ranging from 60% for stage 1 to 5% for stage 4.

Spontaneous remission and regression of metastases following surgical resection of the primary tumour are both recognized but are very rare.

Current issues

Biological therapy for RCC is still being evaluated for metastatic and adjuvant settings. Newer therapies, including gene therapy, are being considered.

Further reading

Long G. Renal cell carcinoma. *Current Opinion in Oncology,* 1997; **9:** 301–6.

Related topics of interest

Biological therapy (p. 7)
Immunotherapy (p. 119)
Interleukin-2 (p. 123)

SARCOMA

Soft tissue sarcomas are a heterogeneous group of rare malignancies, which arise in non-osseous connective tissue. The variety of cell origins is reflected by the wide range of malignancies that arise and the histological appearances.

Incidence
Soft tissue sarcomas are rare cancers with around 1000 new cases per year in the UK. Soft tissue sarcomas occur predominantly in old age but are one of the more common malignancies of adolescence and young adulthood, accounting for less than 1% of adult tumours but approximately 7% of cancer in people under 15 years old.

Risk factors
The Li–Fraumeni syndrome includes soft tissue sarcomas. Other inherited syndromes such as tuberous sclerosis and neurofibromatosis are also associated with an increase of soft tissue sarcomas.

Aetiology
The aetiology is largely unknown, but is probably different for each of the different histological types. Viruses (EBV) and chemical carcinogens have been implicated but not proven as causes. Radiation is recognized as a cause with soft tissue sarcomas occurring within radiation fields several years after treatment.

Chromosome abnormalities have been seen in several sarcomas for example t(2:13) (q37;q14) in alveolar rhabdomyosarcomas and t (11;22)(q24;q12) in peripheral neuroepithelioma.

Single gene defects can also be associated with a genetic predisposition to sarcoma, for example the Li–Fraumeni syndrome of germline *p53* mutation can lead to sarcomas.

Histology
The different histological types reflect the hetereogeneous tissues derived from mesenchymal tissue. For clinical management, soft tissue sarcomas can usefully be divided into low-, intermediate- and high-grade malignancies based on histological features. The more common tumours include:

1. Fibrosarcoma (20–30%). These are intermediate- to high-grade tumours.

2. *Liposarcoma (10–20%).* These arise in adipose tissue and depending on differentiation can be low or high grade.

3. *Rhabdomyosarcoma (15%).* These arise from skeletal muscle and include three categories: embryonal (more common in childhood), alveolar and pleomorphic (more common in adults). These are all high-grade, aggressive tumours.

4. *Leiomyosarcomas (5%).* These arise from smooth muscle and can occur virtually anywhere, but more commonly in the uterus, GI tract and retroperitoneum. They can be low- or high-grade.

Other rarer types include: synovial sarcomas, neurofibrosarcomas, angiosarcomas and Kaposi's sarcoma, alveolar soft part sarcomas.

Clinical features

Presentation

Approximately 60% present in the extremities, 30% in the trunk and 10% in the head and neck region. Soft tissue sarcomas in the extremities usually present as a painless, enlarging soft tissue swelling. Retroperitoneal tumours often present late with back pain. Between 10 and 20% of patients will have detectable metastases at presentation, most commonly in the lung.

Investigations

Staging for distant metastases, in particular for liver and lung metastases, is now usually performed with CT. Pre-operative assessment of local extent is performed with MRI, which gives more defined views of tissue planes.

Histological confirmation is usually with a biopsy, either by needle biopsy or by open incisional or excisional biopsy. This should be done in consultation with a specialist surgeon so that spread across tissue planes during biopsy is minimal and definitive surgery is not compromised.

Staging

There is no widely accepted staging for all the soft tissue sarcomas. Most staging systems take into account histological grade, site, size, spread across tissue planes and distant spread.

Management

Management of soft tissue sarcomas should be co-ordinated through a multi-disciplinary team of reconstructive surgeons, radiotherapists and medical oncologists.

Surgery

The aim of surgery is radical resection with an adequate margin. This specialized surgical procedure must be carried out by an experienced surgeon and support team. Approaches vary but will commonly include resection of an entire anatomical compartment and the origin and insertion of involved muscles. Intracapsular excision is not adequate. Even with such treatments there is a local relapse rate of approximately 20% and a distant relapse rate of approximately 30%. For high-grade tumours radical excision is usually combined with adjuvant radiotherapy and chemotherapy. This, along with improved reconstructive techniques, has resulted in limb sparing surgery becoming more common.

Excision of solitary metastatic disease, for example lung metastases should be considered in lower grade soft tissue sarcomas. Cure may be possible with isolated lesions.

Chemotherapy

Adjuvant chemotherapy may be used in high-grade sarcomas following excision. The benefits of adjuvant chemotherapy still need to be conclusively proven. Active agents include doxorubicin, methotrexate, dacarbazine, ifosfamide and vincristine.

For advanced disease, chemotherapy has response rates ranging from less than 20% to greater than 80%, depending on tumour type. Embryonal rhabdomyosarcomas respond well to aggressive combination chemotherapy. Single agent doxorubicin has a response rate of approximately 15–30% in the majority of adult soft tissue sarcomas, and is the preferred treatment currently.

Radiotherapy

Adjuvant radiotherapy should be given after radical excision of high grade soft tissue sarcomas. High-dose radiation of at least 60 gray is usually used.

For unresectable retroperitoneal tumours radiotherapy can be used to give local control.

Radiotherapy to sites of bony metastases can have a very useful palliative effect.

Prognostic factors

The overall 5 year disease-free survival rates are in the region of 60% for soft tissue sarcomas but vary from approximately 10–95% depending on histological type and stage.

Important prognostic factors are:

- Type of tumour and histological grade.
- Site (extremity better than trunk) because of resection ability.
- Size.
- Distant metastases.
- Age older than 60 associated with a poorer prognosis.

Current issues

- Molecular diagnostics: the application molecular biology techniques to classify and characterize sarcomas (e.g. the presence of certain translocations).
- The use of limb perfusions for soft tissue sarcomas in the periphery.

Related topic of interest

Familial cancer syndromes (p. 92)
Uterine cancer (p. 278)

SCREENING – PRINCIPLES

The identification of early stage disease allows more effective, potentially curative treatment to be used. As early stage disease is frequently asymptomatic, screening may be used to identify tumours before clinical presentation.

Screening tests

Certain characterisitics of both screening test and the tumour should be satisfied.

Tumour

Certain tumour characteristics make them more suitable for screening. Tumours should ideally:

- Be curable when detected early in the majority of the patients.
- Be relatively common.
- Have a long pre-invasive or non-metastatic stage.
- Be able to be detected by relatively simple tests.
- Be distinct from benign lesions.

Test

The ideal screening test would:

- Be able to detect cancer at an early enough stage to implement effective treatment.
- Be sensitive – i.e. able to distinguish tumours clearly and give a low false negative value.
- Be specific – i.e. not giving false positive results.
- Be well tolerated, hence improving compliance.
- Be easy to administer or perform.
- Be inexpensive.
- Be well publicized in order to ensure high uptake amongst the target population.

No ideal screening test exists.

1. *Advantages.* Advantages of screening include:

- Reduction of mortality by detecting early disease that is curable.
- Less radical treatment hence reducing morbidity.
- Saving on health service resources.
- Reassurance given by a negative test.

2. *Disadvantages.* Potential disadvantages include:

- Increased length of anxiety and morbidity if no effective intervention is possible.
- The over-investigation of false positive cases with associated morbidity.
- Over-treatment of borderline cases that do not require treatment.
- False reassurance from a false negative result.
- Possible harmful effects of the screening test.
- Cost of screening a large population.

Cancer screening programmes

There are several ways to reconcile the above factors to achieve useful screening programmes.

- Limit the screening to at-risk populations. This improves the overall sensitivity and specificity. It also often allows more effective targeting of the test and increases compliance. The resource issues are also favourably affected.
- Develop an effective infrastructure, for example through primary health care teams, support groups and through work places to increase awareness and uptake of at-risk populations.

The programmes in place and under evaluation in the UK include:

Cervical cancer
The most effective screening programme up to date. All women aged between 20 and 64 are offered screening every 5 years. Screening every 3 years further reduces the incidence of invasive carcinomas. This is particularly successful because of the relatively long pre-invasive period during which early detection can occur, and an effective treatment for early disease.

Breast cancer
Regular mammography is offered to all women between 50 and 64 year old every 3 years. The ability of mammography to reduce mortality is controversial. Screening for younger patients who are at increased risk, such as those with a family history, should be considered.

Colorectal cancer
The role of faecal occult blood testing or annual flexible sigmoidoscopies for the general population over 50–60 years old is being investigated. At-risk patients, such as those with ulcerative colitis, a strong family history or a

previous primary tumour should be screened with regular colonoscopies. The cost/benefit balance is probably against using such a test in a wider population.

Current issues

Ovarian cancer   Screening of both at-risk patients, that is those with a strong family history, and the general population with CA125 and trans-vaginal ultrasound is being studied.

Prostate cancer   The detection of pre-clinical disease with prostate specific antigen (PSA) and trans-rectal ultrasound is controversial, as the clinical relevance of such disease is unclear.

Genetic screening   Advances in molecular biology has allowed testing for predisposition to various cancers. The ethics of such testing is being debated in many forums. The identification of at-risk populations may allow screening of a more selected population making such screening programmes more effective overall.

Related topics of interest

SMOKING

The WHO estimates that world-wide, tobacco kills more than 3 million people each year. In the UK, cigarette smoking leads to more than 100,000 premature deaths, and is associated with 30% of all cancer deaths. Lifelong smokers have a 50% chance of dying from tobacco-related diseases. Smoking 20 cigarettes per day leads to a 15-year reduction in life expectancy.

Epidemiology

The epidemiological evidence of an association between cigarettes and cancer includes:

- The higher incidence of cancer in smokers compared with non-smokers, i.e. an increased relative risk.
- The reduction in risk seen in ex-smokers compared with those who continue to smoke.
- A clear dose response effect, i.e. an increased risk of cancer is associated with the number of cigarettes smoked per day, years of smoking, age of starting, degree of inhalation, tar/nicotine content.

Smoking-related illnesses

Smoking causes more premature deaths from non-malignant causes than from cancer.

Non-malignant

Cigarette smoking is clearly associated with heart disease (UK smokers aged 30–50 are five times more likely to have a myocardial infarction than non-smokers), cerebrovascular disease, peripheral vascular disease, chronic obstructive airways disease, low birth-weight babies and is a probable cause of peptic ulcer disease, unsuccessful pregnancies and increased infant mortality, including sudden infant death syndrome.

Malignant

Tobacco is believed to be the major aetiological factor in approximately 1 in 3 malignancies. This exceeds other aetiological factors, such as diet (30%), infection (9%), hormones (7%), occupational (3%), radiation (3%) and alcohol (3%).

The malignancies with the clearest association with cigarette smoking include:

1. *Lung.* 85–90% of lung cancer is related to cigarette smoking. In life-long non-smokers the incidence is

10–15 per 100 000, in 20-per-day smokers the risk is 25 times greater. All histological sub-types are increased with smoking, especially squamous, small cell and large cell. Adenocarcinoma is more frequent in smokers but the association is much weaker. Other aetiological agents may act synergistically with cigarette smoking, for example asbestos exposure.

2. *Bladder*. Approximately 50–85% of cases are associated with smoking. There is a 2.5-fold increase in relative risk in an individual smoking 20-per-day. Atypical cells are found in 4% of non-smokers' bladders but in up to 50% of smokers' bladders. The urine of smokers is directly mutagenic to salmonella (Ames test).

3. *Oral cavity, larynx, oesophagus*. Cigarette smoking is a major independent risk factor but also shows a synergistic effect with alcohol. Tumours are rare in the absence of both risk factors.

4. *Stomach*. Smoking is implicated, especially in tumours in the cardia of the stomach.

5. *Pancreas*. Smoking remains the only clearly defined risk factor and is associated with a 2–3-fold increase in relative risk.

6. *Cervical*. A clear association can be demonstrated with cigarette smoking. However whether this is causative rather than a social correlation with other factors such as human papilloma virus (HPV) infection is unclear.

7. *Others*. Renal, liver and brain tumours have been demonstrated in some studies to be associated with cigarette smoking. Other tumours such as breast and colon cancer show no clear correlation.

Carcinogenic properties of cigarettes

Tobacco smoke contains more than 3000 chemicals which may act as carcinogens able to both initiate and promote tumour development. Analysis of DNA from lung and cervical tissue of smokers has demonstrated DNA adducts, covalent bonds between DNA strands which lead to misreplication and mutation.

Carcinogens

The major classes of carcinogens identified in cigarette smoke include:

Polycyclic hydrocarbons. Benzo(a)pyrene is converted to an active metabolite which has been demonstrated *in vivo* to produce DNA adducts at the precise location of the most frequent *p53* mutations seen in lung cancer.

Nitrosamines and aromatic amines. The metabolism of these carcinogens shows considerable inter-individual variability related to the genetic polymorphism of genes such as cytochrome p450 and glutathione S-transferases. This may explain the different response of individuals to a similar carcinogenic insult.

Smoking prevention

Smoking remains the single largest cause of avoidable premature death. Stopping smoking produces major health benefits. One year after quitting, coronary heart disease risk decreases by 50%, and after 15 years risks approach that of non-smoker. Risks of developing lung cancer, obstructive airways disease and stroke decrease more slowly. 10–14 years after stopping smoking the risk of mortality from cancer decreases to that of lifelong non-smokers. Therefore, every effort should be made to encourage patients to stop smoking.

Current issues

Recent legal battles in the USA have resulted in some tobacco companies accepting that nicotine is addictive and that cigarettes cause cancer. Payments of more than £200 billion will be made over 25 years. In the UK, legal aid has recently been withdrawn from former smokers seeking compensation from tobacco companies.

Related topics of interest

Aetiological agents (p. 1)
Lung cancer (p. 136)

STAGING – TNM CLASSIFICATION

The TNM classification accurately defines the stage of a cancer with respect to the primary tumour (T), associated nodal disease (N) and distant metastases (M). This staging system has been accepted by the International Union Against Cancer (UICC) and the American Joint Committee on Cancer (AJCC) to ensure world-wide acceptance of a single staging system.

The role of the TNM classification

A single staging system adopted universally by clinicians allows the exchange and comparison of information between different treatment centres. This enables a clinician to be guided in the management of any individual by the published results of other patients. Survival analysis of different TNM subgroups enables prospective prognostic information to be given to a patient.

TNM staging classification

The TNM system is based upon the anatomical extent of disease of three components. If determined microscopically from pathological specimens it is referred to as the pTNM stage. If determined clinically from physical, radiological, endoscopic or surgical examination it is referred to as the TNM stage (or cTNM).

1. T (tumour). This defines the extent of the primary tumour.

- Tx   Primary tumour cannot be assessed.
- T0   No evidence of primary tumour.
- Tis   Carcinoma *in situ.*
- T1–4   Primary tumour of increasing size and/or location.

The precise definition of T1–T4 incorporates those anatomical features which define prognostic groups and is therefore different for different tumour types. For example, the prognosis of breast tumours is partly related to the size of the primary tumour; a T1 breast tumour is therefore defined as one less than 2 cm in maximum diameter. In contrast the prognosis of bladder carcinomas is partly determined by the depth of invasion; a T1 bladder tumour is therefore defined as one invading only subepithelial connective tissues.

2. *N (nodes)*. This defines the absence or presence and extent of regional lymph node metastases. This includes the direct invasion of a lymph node by a primary tumour.

Nx   Regional lymph nodes cannot be assessed.
N0   No regional lymph node metastases.
N1–3 Define increasing lymph node involvement.

The definition of N1–N3 again relates to the pattern of nodal disease and its relationship to prognosis for each primary tumour. N1 breast cancer defines mobile ipsilateral axillary lymph nodes, N1 bladder cancer defines a single nodal metastasis less than 2 cm in its greatest diameter.

3. *M (metastases)*. This defines the absence or presence of distant metastases.

Mx   Distant metastases cannot be assessed.
M0   No distant metastases.
M1   Distant metastases present.

The M1 stage is sub-classified by the site of metastasis (i.e. M1(PUL) refers to pulmonary metastases, M1(BRA) refers to brain metastases). The M staging is therefore consistent for all diseases.

Stage grouping

The T, N, and M definitions allow precise allocation of stage into 24 possible subgroups. More simple classifications have been devised for many diseases which group patients of different TNM subgroup but similar prognosis into a single stage group (e.g. Dukes' classification of colon cancer):

Stage A: confined to the bowel wall [i.e. mucosa and submucosa, or early muscular invasion (T1–2, N0, M0)].
Stage B: invasion through the muscle wall but no lymph node involvement (T3, N0, M0).
Stage C: lymph node involvement (any T, N1–3, M0).
Stage D: distant metastases or advanced local disease (any T, any N, M1 or T4).

Inadequate staging

An accurate staging system greatly enhances the management of cancer patients. However, inaccurate staging within such a system has significant consequences and generally occurs as the result of inadequate staging procedures. An endoscopic biopsy is rarely able to define the final staging of the primary tumour as full thickness biopsies are not performed. Inadequate radiological assessment may fail to identify pulmonary or brain metastases. This means that patients may be under staged (i.e. they are assigned to a stage lower than their true status). This in turn affects survival statistics.

Further reading

UICC. In: Hermanek P, Sobin LH, eds. *TNM Classification of Malignant Tumours*, 4th edn. Berlin: Springer, 1992.

SURGICAL ONCOLOGY – PRINCIPLES

Most cancer patients will require surgical intervention. This may be an initial diagnostic biopsy, a potentially curative resection of a solid tumour or a palliative procedure.

Diagnosis

A tissue diagnosis is virtually mandatory in all patients and often requires direct biopsy of the lesion. Many forms of biopsy are available including fine-needle aspiration cytology, Tru-Cut needle biopsy, incisional and excisional biopsy. Ideally the biopsy should be performed by an experienced surgeon who will be involved in the definitive tumour resection. The surgeon should also be familiar with the most suitable biopsy technique for any particular tumour site and type. The positioning of the biopsy should not jeopardise the final margins of tumour clearance or any possible reconstructive procedure. The surgeon should have access to experienced cytologists, histopathologists and radiologists to confirm the diagnosis.

Tumour staging

Staging allows selection of the most appropriate management for an individual patient. Despite the accuracy of modern imaging techniques, surgery still has a role in the assessment of stage in some malignancies. For example, axillary node dissection in patients with breast cancer is vital to accurately assess the presence and degree of metastatic disease thereby defining the risk of future relapse and the need for further treatment.

Laparoscopy and thoracoscopy may allow more accurate staging and assessment of the resectability of a tumour and avoid the morbidity of a laparotomy or thoracotomy in patients with unresectable cancer.

Tumour resection

Approximately a third of cancer patients are potentially curable by surgery alone. Patients can be cured if their tumour is localized, with limited spread to regional nodes or with resectable metastases. Cure and local recurrence rates are surgeon-dependent which emphasizes the need for specialist care. Resection of a primary tumour optimizes the conditions required to eradicate distant micrometastases with chemotherapy.

Lymph nodes	Resection of regional lymph nodes may provide staging information and reduce the incidence of disease relapse in the nodes. In some tumours, lymph node resection confers a survival advantage. However, the benefits must be considered against the possible morbidity of the procedure such as lymphoedema and associated nerve damage. The role of radical procedures to dissect more distant lymph nodes has in some situations been shown to adversely affect survival, for example in bladder cancer. Its role in any setting should be carefully assessed within controlled trials.
Metastases	The resection of distant metastases is most commonly performed in patients with hepatic metastases from colorectal primaries. Metastases suitable for resection are generally single or confined to a single lobe of the liver. Only 5% of patients with hepatic metastases are suitable but overall 5 year survival is increased from 5% to 25%.
	Resection of isolated brain or lung metastases in various tumours have also produced clinical cures or prolonged disease-free periods. A thorough pre-operative search for other lesions is obviously required in these patients.
Recurrent disease	Recurrent disease at the primary site can, uncommonly, be cured by a secondary resection in some cancers, including colorectal cancer. The resection of recurrent disease also has a definite place in symptom control where, in conjunction with chemotherapy or radiotherapy, it can provide a worthwhile period of remission.

Palliative surgery

Palliative surgery is only indicated where an improvement in the patient's quality of life is likely. The distress of a hospital stay and surgical procedure must also be considered against possible benefit.

Tumour resection	Local resection of a tumour, irrespective of distant metastatic disease, may provide local control and freedom from associated symptoms. Resection of a stenosing colorectal primary in the presence of liver metastases may prevent the morbidity and mortality associated with an acute obstruction.

Symptom control

Haemorrhage. Persisting haematuria from an unresectable tumour can be controlled with arterial embolization.

Dysphagia. Palliation may be achieved with endoscopically placed stents, re-establishing the lumen of the oesophagus by laser resection or alcohol injections into the tumour.

Gastrointestinal obstruction. Obstruction of small or large bowel due to a locally unresectable tumour is nearly always relieved by a bypass procedure. Endoscopic or radiological stenting now provides an alternative method of overcoming colorectal obstruction. Bowel obstruction due to diffuse peritoneal or intra-abdominal cancer is rarely relieved by an operation and medical management may provide more appropriate palliative care.

Obstructive jaundice. Biliary obstruction may be alleviated by the use of a stent inserted endoscopically or percutaneously.

Drainage of effusions. Symptomatic ascites or pleural effusions can be relieved by the intermittent insertion of a drainage catheter. In-dwelling shunts may also be appropriate.

Prophylaxis

Patients at high risk of tumour development identified by a strong family history and/or the presence of a genetic marker/gene may be considered for prophylactic surgery. Examples include prophylactic mastectomy for familial breast cancer and total colectomy in people with familial polyposis coli.

Further reading

Baines M. In: Doyle D, Hanks GWC, Macdonald N, eds. *Oxford Textbook of Palliative Medicine.* Oxford University Press, 1996, Chapter 4, part 3.4.

Barr LC, Skene AI, Thomas JM. Metastastectomy. *British Journal of Surgery,* 1992; **79:** 1268–74.

Rosenberg SA. In: DeVita VT, Hellman S, Rosenberg SA, eds. *Cancer: Principles and Practise of Oncology,* 5th edn. Philadelphia: Lippincott-Raven, 1997, Chapter 15.

TAMOXIFEN

Tamoxifen is the most widely used hormonal therapy in current use and has been used for more than 20 years.

Uses

Breast cancer. Tamoxifen is prescribed to most patients with advanced disease and as an adjuvant therapy following primary surgical cancer. In advanced disease the response rate is dependent on the oestrogen receptor status of the tumour. However, in the UK this is not always assessed and most patients are prescribed tamoxifen, with about 1/3 of unselected patients achieving a reponse. Adjuvant therapy with tamoxifen reduces local and distant tumour recurrence, reduces the risk of a second breast primary developing and improves survival following primary surgery.

In elderly patients tamoxifen may be used as the only treatment modality as it has few side effects.

Others. Tamoxifen is also used in the management of melanoma, renal, ovarian and endometrial cancer. Although objective reponses are infrequent, it may provide a useful palliative effect in these tumours.

Mode of action

Tamoxifen acts on tumour cells partly by binding the oestrogen receptor and thus antagonizing oestrogen-mediated growth stimuli. The response rate of advanced disease to tamoxifen is dependent on the receptor status of the tumour. Of those tumours that express both oestrogen and progesterone receptors 77% have been demonstrated to respond to tamoxifen. In those tumours which do not express either receptor a response rate of only 11% has been reported. Its activity against oestrogen receptor-negative tumour cells suggests that other modes of action in addition to its oestrogen antagonism are important.

On some other tissues, tamoxifen acts as a partial oestrogen agonist (e.g. it may have cardioprotective effects and prevent loss of bone mineralization in post-menopausal women).

Pharmacokinetics

Tamoxifen is well absorbed orally and is highly protein-bound in the circulation. It is extensively metabolized to a number of active metabolites and excreted in the bile.

Scheduling	In breast cancer, tamoxifen is generally given as a once daily dose of 20 mg, and is usually commenced immediately post surgery in the adjuvant setting. There is controversy regarding the length of time that a patient should remain on tamoxifen therapy. Current opinion is that up to 5 years is appropriate but there are extensive trials investigating this issue.
Toxicity	Tamoxifen is generally very well tolerated. Mild GI disturbance, skin rashes and menopausal-like symptoms (weight gain, flushing and irregular menstrual periods) are common but rarely disabling. Depression is recognized in a small percentage of patients.

The risk of thromboembolic disease is increased on tamoxifen. However, the risk is no more than that associated with the oral contraceptive pill or hormone replacement therapy.

Secondary malignancies associated with tamoxifen therapy have been documented. However, a large overview of adjuvant tamoxifen therapy demonstrated no increase in secondary malignancies other than those of the endometrium. Endometrial carcinoma has been reported in 23 out of 1372 patients on adjuvant tamoxifen, an increase in relative risk of approximately five-fold. Hepatocellular carcinoma has only been reported in patients receiving high doses of tamoxifen (40 mg bd) and not in those receiving standard doses.

It is vital that the risks of tamoxifen are balanced against the very significant benefits to the patient, not only in the prevention of breast cancer but also in the reduction in cardiovascular mortality and osteoporosis.

Current issues

The optimal duration of adjuvant tamoxifen therapy is unresolved and therefore the focus of clinical studies world-wide.

The role of tamoxifen in preventing breast cancers developing in high-risk women (i.e. those with a strong family history) is being assessed.

Related topic of interest

Breast cancer (p. 30)
Uterine cancer (p. 267)

TAXANES

Paclitaxel (Taxol®) and docetaxel (Taxotere®) are the first two members of a new class of anti-cancer drug, the taxanes. They are natural compounds derived from the yew tree: paclitaxel from the bark of the Pacific yew and docetaxel from the needles of the European yew. This has made the taxanes difficult and therefore costly to manufacture.

Uses

Paclitaxel is licensed in the UK for the treatment of metastatic ovarian cancer where standard platinum-based therapy has failed. However, both paclitaxel and docetaxel are being widely investigated in a wide range of solid malignancies. Their use in the treatment of metastatic breast, bladder and lung cancer (both SCLC and NSCLC) is established within the context of clinical trials and studies. Their use has been investigated both as therapy for disease resistant to conventional treatment and as first-line agents either in combination with other drugs or as a single agent.

Paclitaxel's primary indication is in the management of ovarian cancer. In patients who have truly platinum-resistant disease a response rate of 25–30% is seen.

Mode of action

The taxanes act by affecting the network of microtubules within a cell. This network forms the structural architecture of the cell and in particular the mitotic spindle, along which the chromosomes separate during the interphase of cell division. The disruption of the dynamic network is believed to be central to its cytotoxicity.

Pharmacokinetics

Paclitaxel is extensively (89%) protein bound within the serum. Its metabolism is predominantly hepatic with minimal renal excretion. Its use in patients with severe hepatic dysfunction is therefore avoided.

Scheduling

Paclitaxel is given in by intravenous infusion, over 3 hours, at doses of approximately 175 mg/m², every 3 weeks. Higher doses or shorter dose intervals can be achieved with the use of growth factor, stem cell or bone marrow support. More prolonged infusions (24 hours) have been given with no convincing increase in efficacy but an increase in toxicity, especially the degree of myelosuppression. Allergic reactions (see below) are greatly reduced with the use of corticosteroids, antihistamines and H_2 antagonists as pre-medication. The adminstration of paclitaxel requires the use of non-PVC-containing equipment as the oil in which the drug is prepared leaches pthalates from PVC.

Toxicity

1.   Myelosupression. This is the dose-limiting toxicity, with approximately 25% of patients experiencing severe neutropenia. Anaemia and thrombocytopenia are less common.

2.   Nausea and vomiting. This is rarely severe and usually well controlled with standard anti-emetics.

3.   Alopecia. This occurs in almost every patient receiving paclitaxel.

4.   Extravasation. Paclitaxel is a moderate vesicant.

5.   Peripheral neuropathy. This commonly presents as paraesthesia in a stocking/glove distribution. Severe (grade 3 or 4) neuropathy warrants dose reduction or stopping of paclitaxel therapy. It tends to improve when paclitaxel is discontinued.

6.   General myalgia and arthralgia. These are very common (~50%) but usually well controlled with non-steroidal analgesia.

7.   Allergic reactions. Both paclitaxel and docetaxel are associated with frequent hypersensitivity reactions on administration.

Current issues

The role of paclitaxel as first-line therapy for ovarian carcinoma is the focus of many studies. A recent study in the USA demonstrated an improved response rate and increased survival in patients who received a combination of paclitaxel and cisplatin compared with those receiving cisplatin and cyclophosphamide. These results require confirmation in current trials such as ICON 3 before the adoption of this therapy as the first-line regime.

Related topic of interest

Ovarian cancer (p. 181)

TESTICULAR CANCER

Testicular tumours are predominantly germ cell tumours. Germ cell tumours may arise at other sites in the body. Testicular germ cell tumours, although highly metastatic, are sensitive to treatment and may frequently be cured.

Background

Incidence

The incidence of testicular cancer is 20 per million of the population with approximately 1500 new cases diagnosed each year in the UK. Predominantly occurring in 20–40 year olds. The incidence is increasing world-wide.

Risk factors

Maldescent of testes predisposes to germ cell tumours.

Aetiology

The pathogenesis of germ cell tumours is unknown. No well characterised genetic changes typical of germ cell tumours have yet been defined.

Histology

Germ cell tumours comprise approximately 90% of testicular tumours, with the remaining 10% being predominantly lymphomas or soft tissue sarcomas. Several histological classifications of testicular germ cell tumours exist:

Seminomas. These account for 40% of cases.

Non-seminomatous germ cell tumours (NSGCT). These account for 60% of cases.

- Malignant teratoma: well differentiated; moderately differentiated; poorly differentiated.
- Combined seminoma/non-seminoma.
- Yolk sac tumours.

Tumours can have a mixed histological appearance.

Early spread is common via lymphatics to para-aortic nodes, reflecting the embryological origin from primitive para-renal tissues. Blood-borne spread to lungs, liver, bone and brain is common in advanced disease.

Clinical features

Presentation

Presentation is usually with localized disease with a painless testicular swelling. Metastatic spread can present with symptoms, for example cough or dyspnoea due to lung metastases, or as low back pain due to para-aortic involvement.

Investigations

Testicular ultrasound will differentiate solid from a fluid-filled masses and is the initial investigation of choice. Features on the ultrasound can also differentiate between teratomas and seminomas.

Tumour markers (βHCG and AFP). β human chorionic gonadotrophin (βHCG) is raised in both seminomas and teratomas in up to 75% of patients. α-Fetoprotein (AFP) is only raised in the presence of teratomatous elements. Lactate dehydrogenase (LDH) is a useful marker to assess prognosis, response to treatment and detect relapse.

Orchidectomy. This is required for tissue diagnosis and as definitive therapy for localized disease. Biopsy of the contralateral testicle is indicated in patients with cryptorchids or a history of testicular maldescent as there is an increased risk of bilateral disease in these situations. Trans-scrotal biopsy is contra-indicated, because of the risk of dissemination of the tumour.

CT. CT scanning of chest, abdomen and pelvis has largely replaced other investigations such as lymphangiography.

Staging

The Royal Marsden staging system is most commonly used:

Stage I: confined to testicle.
Stage II: involving para-aortic lymph nodes below the diaphragm.
Stage III: involving para-aortic lymph nodes above the diaphragm.
Stage IV: involving visceral metastases.

Management

Germ cell tumours are highly malignant with rapid growth and high metastatic potential, but are also generally very sensitive to chemotherapy and radiotherapy. The clinical distinction between a seminoma and a tumour with non-seminomatous elements (NSGCT) determines management.

Surgery

Orchidectomy is required for diagnosis and for definitive treatment of localized disease. This should be performed via the inguinal canal to reduce risk of spread through scrotal tissue planes. Biopsy of the contralateral side is often performed at the time of operation.

In metastatic teratoma, surgery is generally performed for the resection of any residual mass that remains after chemotherapy. Careful examination of the resected mass is required to assess the presence of viable tumour which may necessitate further systemic treatment. Removal is also necessary to prevent regrowth of teratomas and growth of non-germ cell elements which are occasionally present.

Chemotherapy

Both seminomas and teratomas are chemosensitive with response rates of over 90%. Platinum-containing combination chemotherapies are used to treat advanced seminoma (stage III and above) or following relapse after radiotherapy. Chemotherapy with bleomycin, etoposide and cisplatin (BEP) is most frequently used, with 3–4 cycles usually being given. Usual practice is to treat the patient until a complete remission is achieved and then give one more cycle.

Advanced malignant NSGCT (stage II and above) is also treated with BEP chemotherapy. Dose intensity should be maintained if possible and haematopoetic growth factors can be used to aid recovery between courses.

Second-line chemotherapy for relapsed patients include combinations using procarbazine, doxorubicin and alkylating agents (e.g. POM-ACE: procarbazine/vincristine/methotrexate/adriamycin/cyclophosphamide/etoposide).

High-dose chemotherapy with peripheral stem cell support is being assessed increasingly for poor prognosis patients, either as part of initial therapy following induction with conventional dose BEP chemotherapy or on relapse.

Radiotherapy
Radiotherapy to the para-aortic nodes is used in stage I seminomas as adjuvant treatment. Stage II disease is also commonly treated with radiotherapy to the para-aortic nodes. More advanced disease or poorer prognosis disease is treated with chemotherapy.

For malignant teratoma, radiotherapy to sites of bulky metastatic disease is used in conjunction with chemotherapy. Palliative radiotherapy to localized sites such as bone, brain and nodes is often effective.

Prognostic factors

Bulky tumour sites
These carry a worse prognosis.

Histological markers
The presence of yolk sac elements, vascular invasion or lymphatic invasion predict a poorer prognosis.

Tumour markers
Markedly raised AFP, bHCG and LDH are associated with poor prognosis.

An international germ cell tumour prognostic classification has recently been developed based on a retrospective analysis of patients. Groups are divided into good, intermediate and poor prognostic groups depending on site of the primary, visceral metastases (pulmonary metastases have a good prognosis) and levels of tumour markers. Mediastinal primary germ cell tumours carry a uniformly poor prognosis.

Stage I seminoma:	cure rate of greater than 95%.
Stage II seminoma:	cure rate of greater than 70%.
Stage I NSGCT:	cure rate greater than 95%.
Stage II NSGCT:	cure rate greater than 95%.
Stage II NSGCT:	cure rate greater than 95%.
Stage IV NSGCT:	cure rate greater than 50%.

Screening

There is no role at present for routine screening. Self-examination programmes are however being promoted.

Current issues

- Campaigns to increase public awareness of disease and the importance of self-examination are being undertaken.
- The role of high-dose chemotherapy with peripheral blood stem cells is being investigated in poor risk patients.

Related topic of interest

Chemotherapy – (b) combination (p. 52)

THYROID CANCER

Background

Incidence

Thyroid cancer is an uncommon malignancy but is the most frequent endocrine tumour. It accounts for around 1% of all cancers, with approximately 1000 new cases diagnosed each year in the UK. It is more frequent in females, with a ratio of 3:1.

Risk factors

1. *Radiation.* The risk of developing thyroid cancer is directly related to the dose of radiation to which an individual is exposed. Children and females are at particular risk. A latent period of up to 40 years may occur before cancer develops. Children treated with radiotherapy to the head and neck have a lifetime risk of thyroid cancer of 1/16.

2. *TSH stimulation.* Although prolonged TSH stimulation is associated with thyroid cancer in animals, the relationship of thyroid cancer to endemic goitre is unclear.

3. *Familial.* Medullary thyroid cancer occurs as part of the multiple endocrine neoplasia (MEN) syndrome type 2.

Histology

There are four main varieties of thyroid cancer.

1. *Papillary.* 60% of thyroid cancers are differentiated papillary. These tend to be multifocal at presentation. Early metastatic spread via lymphatics is common.

2. *Follicular.* 15% are differentiated follicular. They are unifocal and early spread is typically to bone and lung via the blood. They can be difficult to distinguish histologically from a benign adenoma with atypia.

Papillary and follicular differentiated tumours tend to be extremely slow growing with doubling times of more than 1 year.

3. *Anaplastic.* These tumours tend to occur in older age groups. They present with locally advanced disease and respond poorly to treatment.

4. *Medullary.* These are rare tumours which arise from the parafollicular cells of the thyroid. They can secrete calcitonin which may act as a serum marker of disease. They occur both sporadically (usually unilaterally) and in families (almost always bilaterally) as part of the MEN-2 syndrome.

Other histological types include lymphoma (~5%) and sarcoma.

Clinical features

Presentation

Thyroid cancer invariably presents with a thyroid mass. However, thyroid masses are present in approximately 5% of adults, of which only 5–20 % are due to malignancy.

Investigations

1. *Thyroid scan.* The uptake of radiolabelled iodine or technetium may be used to assess the mass. A cold nodule represents a malignancy in up to 15% although the frequency increases in patients under 40. Less than 1% of hot nodules are due to cancer.

2. *Biopsy.* Fine needle aspiration cytology is generally adequate to diagnose a malignant lesion. Benign cysts may also be identified and drained.

3. *Ultrasound.* This is unable to distinguish between a benign and malignant lesion although may identify a thyroid cyst.

4. *Thyroid function tests.* These are usually normal.

5. *Thyroglobulin monitoring.* This is rarely useful in the management but may occasionally be raised.

Staging

Thyroid cancer is staged with the TNM classification.

Management

Surgery

Primary treatment is surgical excision biopsy of the mass. The extent of surgery is controversial in limited disease. Total thyroidectomy avoids the 5–10% recurrence rate associated with lobectomy but is associated with a significantly higher rate of complications (hypoparathyroidism and laryngeal nerve palsy). Patients at high risk of recurrence should receive a near total or total thyroidectomy. Abnormal regional lymph nodes should be biopsied at initial surgery but radical lymph node dissection is not indicated

Endocrine therapy

All patients should receive thyroxine to suppress the TSH level without inducing clinical thyrotoxicosis. This reduces the rate of recurrence and should be maintained if possible.

Radiotherapy

I^{131}. In differentiated tumours limited to the thyroid, the use of radiolabelled iodine has reduced the rate of recurrence in some studies but its use is not routine. In locally advanced or metastatic disease, I^{131} may be given to ablate the residual tumour if this is demonstrated to take up the isotope.

External beam irradiation. Tumours which are irresectable and do not bind iodine may be treated with external beam radiotherapy.

Chemotherapy

Doxorubicin and bleomycin are the most active single agents with response rates of approximately 30%. Combination regimes containing these drugs may improve response rates. However, response durations are short and therefore chemotherapy is rarely used.

Prognostic factors

Histology

- Papillary: 95% 10 year survival.
- Follicular: 90% 10 year survival.
- Medullary: 40% 10 year survival.
- Anaplastic: 5% 10 year survival.

Stage	Large primary tumours, extrathyroid extension and distant metastases adversely effect prognosis. The 5 year survival of patients with distant metastases is 22%.
	The prognostic significance of lymph nodes metastases is controversial with conflicting evidence from different studies.
Patient demographics	Female gender and younger age are associated with a favourable prognosis.

Current issues

Detection of individuals with an increased risk of thyroid carcinoma by genetic screening for MEN syndromes.

Further reading

Tubiana M, Shumberger M. In: Peckham M, Pinedo H, Veroneri U, eds. *Oxford Textbook of Oncology*. Oxford University Press, 1995; 2097–2122.

Related topic of interest

Endocrine tumours (p. 83)

TUMOUR MARKERS

Tumour markers are substances produced either by or in response to a tumour, which are present in blood or other tissue fluids and can be quantified.

- Sensitivity. The sensitivity of a marker relates to its ability to detect those with a certain disease. If 100 people have the disease and the marker is elevated in only 95, its sensitivity is 0.95.
- Specificity. The specificity of a marker relates to its ability to accurately define those who are disease free. If in 100 disease-free people the marker is negative in only 90 (i.e. there are 10 false positives) the specificity of the test is 0.90.

A tumour marker therefore should be both highly sensitive so that few people with the disease are missed *and* highly specific so that few people are falsely labelled as having the disease.

Classes

- Cell-surface glycoproteins: carcino-embryonic antigen (CEA), CA125, CA19.9.
- Oncofetal proteins: β human chorionic gonadotrophin (βHCG), α-fetoprotein (AFP).
- Enzymes: acid phosphatase, alkaline phosphatase, lactate dehydrogenase, neurone-specific enolase.
- Inorganic molecules: calcium, phosphate, sodium.
- Intermediate metabolites: 5-hydroxyindoleacetic acid, vanillyl mandelic acid.
- Hormones: thyroglobulin, antidiuretic hormone, adrenocorticotrophic hormone.
- Immunoglobulins: Bence–Jones protein.
- Cytokines and their receptors.
- Nucleic acids: both DNA and RNA can be detected. These can be tumour-specific (e.g. Philadelphia chromosome, oncogene mutations), or tissue-specific [e.g. the detection of tyrosinase expression (a melanocyte-specific gene) in blood].

Uses

Screening

The use of existing tumour markers to screen the general population cannot currently be justified. Their use has not yet been shown to alter clinical outcome in randomized controlled trials. However certain high risk groups have been identified in whom screening can be justified (e.g. the use of AFP to detect the development of hepatocellular carcinoma in patients with cirrhosis caused by chronic viral hepatitis).

Diagnosis

Under some circumstances, tumour markers can be very helpful in diagnosis but most are elevated in a broad spectrum of malignancies (e.g. CEA, initially thought to be specific for colorectal carcinoma, is elevated in a proportion of patients with pancreatic, gastric, breast and lung malignancies and by smoking). Many are elevated in benign conditions, CA125 for example is elevated in endometriosis, menstruation and pregnancy. A proportion of normal individuals have what has been classified as an 'abnormal' level, 1% of normal women have a CA125 level greater than 35 U/ml. However, within these constraints tumour markers may be of use in diagnosis of a malignancy, particularly in the patient with a malignancy of unknown primary origin. For example prostate-specific antigen (PSA) is highly tissue specific and a marked elevation in a patient with disseminated malignancy is usually diagnostic of prostatic carcinoma. As levels increase certain tumour markers become more suggestive of a particular malignancy. In a series of 888 women a CA125 level greater than 200 U/ml was diagnostic of ovarian malignancy. AFP levels greater than 500 ng/ml are associated only with hepatocellular carcinoma or germ cell tumours.

Prognosis

Certain tumour markers can give an indication of a patient's prognosis. In testicular teratoma, concentrations of βHCG or AFP are powerful determinants of outcome. The rate of decline of a tumour marker post surgery or other treatments has also been shown to relate to prognosis and may influence subsequent management.

Staging

Tumour markers give indirect indication of stage in certain tumours. PSA levels less than 10 ng/ml imply no extracapsular spread and therefore further staging investigations are considered unnecessary.

Response

One of the most clinically useful features of tumour markers is their ability to indicate response to treatment. In a patient with an elevated tumour marker, a reduction in the level of that marker whilst receiving treatment is highly suggestive of a response. The speed of reduction in βHCG and AFP following chemotherapy for germ cell tumours has been demonstrated to relate directly to survival.

Relapse

In a patient who has previously been demonstrated to be marker positive, subsequent increase in the level is highly suggestive of tumour relapse. However, many tumours when relapsing will not show a rise in marker levels and therefore over-reliance on a persistently normal level is dangerous.

Common tumour markers

CEA

This is elevated in a wide variety of tumours but its common clinical use is in the setting of colorectal carcinoma. The occurrence and degree of elevation is related to the clinical stage (4% in Dukes' stage A, 65% with Dukes' stage D) and also correlates with the presence of vascular invasion. It is a cell-surface antigen also expressed in a variety of normal tissues. Ninety-eight per cent of normal non-smokers have levels less than 5 ng/ml. Elevated levels are also more common in smokers, inflammatory bowel disease, hepatitis, pancreatitis and gastritis.

CA125

This is used as a marker of ovarian carcinoma, and is an antigen that is expressed on the surface of ovarian cells. An elevated serum level (≥35 U/ml) has been found in 1% of normal women, 6% with benign conditions (pregnancy, endometriosis and pelvic inflammatory disease) and 82% of women with ovarian carcinoma. Levels greater than 65 U/ml have been observed in 0.2% of normal women, 2% with benign conditions and 73% with ovarian carcinoma. A level greater than 200 U/ml was not found in normal women or those with benign conditions. As with most markers its elevation is not specific for one tumour. Serum levels are also elevated in pancreatic (59%), lung (32%), colorectal (21%) and breast cancer (12%).

AFP

AFP is a glycoprotein produced by the normal fetal yolk sac, liver and intestines. It is undetectable in normal individuals after the first year of life. Its level is moderately elevated in hepatitis but high levels are also produced by hepatocellular carcinoma and cancers containing yolk sac elements (e.g. teratoma). High levels of AFP predict a poor prognosis.

HCG

A glycoprotein consisting of two subunits. HCG is elevated in patients with gestational trophoblastic disease (hydatiform mole, invasive mole, choriocarcinoma). There is also a specific elevation of the β subunit in patients with non-seminomatous testicular cancers and in a small minority of those with seminoma. It is also raised in pregnancy!

Immunoglobulins

These can be a measure of the paraproteinaemias (e.g. myeloma and Waldenstrom's macroglobulinaemia) and occasionally non-Hodgkin's lymphoma. They can be measured in the blood or their excretion can be measured as light chains in the urine (Bence–Jones protein), which occurs in 40–50% of all cases of myeloma.

Current issues

- The identification of new tumour markers detected by more sensitive methods such as PCR.
- Studies examining the use of PSA, CA125 and other markers are currently running to assess the feasibility of these tests as screening tools in the general population.

Related topics of interest

Colrectal cancer (p. 71)
Primary unknown (cancer of unknown origin) (p. 205)

UTERINE CANCER

Background

Incidence

Carcinoma of the endometrial lining of the uterus is a relatively frequent gynaecological malignancy with approximately 4000 new cases per year in the UK. Although predominantly a disease of elderly post-menopausal women, 20% occur in younger women. The incidence appears to be rising, particularly in younger women.

Risk factors

Risk factors include age, menopause, obesity, low parity, early menarche and late menopause. It is associated with excess oestrogen exposure, either endogenous or exogenous. Tamoxifen is associated with a small increased risk of endometrial cancer.

Aetiology

Excess oestrogen exposure may lead to the development of endometrial hyperplasia. Subsequent dysplastic change may lead to carcinoma.

Uterine leiomyosarcomas may result from malignant change in a uterine leiomyoma (fibroid).

Histology

Ninety percent of uterine tumours are endometrial carcinomas. These include:

- Endometrioid adenocarcinoma (more than 75%).
- Mucinous carcinoma.
- Serous carcinoma (less than 10%).
- Squamous carcinomas (occur rarely).

Other tumours include

- Uterine leiomyosarcomas.
- Endometrial stromal sarcomas.
- Mixed mesodermal tumours (contain both epithelial and mesenchymal components).

Clinical features

Presentation

Post menopausal bleeding is the most common presenting feature. Pain is not a common feature. In perimenopausal women, intermenstrual bleeding frequently occurs.

Investigations

Diagnosis is by curettage of the endocervix and the endometrial cavity. Examination under anaesthesia should also be performed. An enlarged uterine corpus suggests myometrial involvement although it may be due to coexistent benign pathology. Ultrasound or CT scans may provide accurate measurements of uterine size and evaluate depth of invasion.

Staging

The International Federation of Gynaecology and Obstetrics (FIGO) staging is as follows:

Stage 0:   Carcinoma *in situ.*
Stage 1:   Carcinoma confined to the corpus uteri.
    1a: Uterine cavity 8 cm or less in length.
    1b: Uterine cavity greater than 8 cm.
Stage 2:   Extension to cervix only.
Stage 3:   Extension beyond the uterus but disease confined to the true pelvis.
Stage 4:   Extension beyond true pelvis, or invasion of bladder or rectum.

Management

Surgery

Total abdominal hysterectomy and bilateral salpingo-oophorectomy is the treatment of choice for localized disease.

Radiotherapy

Endometrial carcinoma is a radiosensitive malignancy. Radiation can be delivered either by the intracavity or the external beam methods.

Radiotherapy is frequently combined with surgery in the management of localized disease. It is of particular use in those patients with poorly differentiated tumours or myometrial invasion, in whom recurrence is more frequent. Neoadjuvant radiotherapy may be used in some patients prior to surgical resection.

In patients with advanced disease, radiotherapy may be used as an alternative to surgery.

Endocrine therapy

Disseminated endometrial cancer is best treated with progestogen therapy. There is a response rate of about

35% and this is associated with prolonged survival. Medroxyprogesterone acetate is given orally and is generally well tolerated.

Chemotherapy   In patients who progress on progesterone therapy, chemotherapy may be of value. Activity in endometrial carcinoma has been demonstrated with single agent adriamycin or cisplatin. Other active drugs include 5-FU, cyclophosphamide, vincristine and doxorubicin.

Prognostic factors

Stage of disease   Stage 1: >75% 5 year survival.
Stage 2: 60% 5 year survival.
Stage 3: 30% 5 year survival.
Stage 4: 10% 5 year survival.

Myometrial invasion   For localized disease the depth of myometrial invasion is related to prognosis.

Screening

There is no screening procedure for cancer of the endometrium. All women with post-menopausal bleeding should have appropriate investigation with endometrial curretage.

Current issues

Tamoxifen   Tamoxifen is now widely used in women following treatment for breast carcinoma. Two years of tamoxifen therapy 20 mg per day has been associated with a relative risk of endometrial carcinoma twice that of the rest of the population. These risks need to be weighed against the benefit of 2 years of tamoxifen therapy in reducing the risk of contralateral breast carcinoma by 29%.

Related topics of interest

Sarcoma (p. 234)
Tamoxifen (p. 250)

VINCRISTINE AND VINBLASTINE

The vinca alkaloids, vincristine, vinblastine and vindesine are both naturally occuring chemotherapeutic agents derived from the perrywinkle. They are prescribed widely in the treatment of both solid and haematological malignancies as part of combination regimes.

Uses

Vincristine and vinblastine are used in the treatment of the leukaemias, lymphomas, paediatric solid tumours, soft-tissue sarcomas and bladder, breast and lung carcinomas.

Vincristine is occasionally prescribed in idiopathic thrombocytopenic purpura refractory to other treatments.

Mode of action

The vinca alkaloids act by disrupting the formation of the mitotic spindle and other components of the cytoskeleton. This disrupts cell division and principally affects and holds the cell at the S phase of the cell cycle.

Pharmacokinetics

The vinca alkaloids are extensively protein-bound in the serum. Their excretion is predominantly hepatic and therefore administration in patients with hepatic dysfunction requires additional caution.

Scheduling

Vincristine and vinblastine are both given as bolus injections. Their administration is dominated by their profound vesicant nature and they must therefore be given into a large vein with a fast flowing drip. The vinca alkaloids are usually given on a weekly schedule, but may be infused over a few days.

Toxicity

1. *Myelosuppression.* Vincristine does not cause myelosuppression and is therefore a useful addition to a combination of other myelosuppressive drugs. A reactive thrombocytosis may occur following administration and therefore vincristine is occasionally given specificially to improve the platelet counts in patients with impaired marrow function. Vinblastine is moderately myelosuppressive.

2. *Gastrointestinal.* Vincristine and vinblastine are both only mildly emetogenic and rarely cause clinically

significant problems. Constipation and colicky abdominal pains occasionally occur. With continued use, a GI ileus may occur.

3. Alopecia. Alopecia is uncommon and rarely total.

4. Extravasation. The vinca alkaloids are the most vesicant chemotherapeutic drugs administered. Extravasation will cause significant burns that may require skin grafts, and therefore the preparation and administration of the vinca alkaloids should be done with extreme care and by trained personnel. If extravasation does occur prompt treatment is essential including extensive lavage, hydrocortisone injections and S/C administration of hyaluronidase. A plastic surgery opinion should be sought early with a view to open lavage of the area.

5. Neurotoxicity. A peripheral, predominantly sensory, neuropathy is the dose-limiting toxicity of vincristine and limits the dose to a maximum of 2 mg per week in all patients. A dose reduction is usually required in the elderly and other patients at risk of developing a peripheral neuropathy such as diabetics. Neuritic pain and subjective parasthesia affect many patients. Cerebellar and cerebral toxicity are rarely seen with either drug. The neurotoxicity of the vinca alkaloids is usually reversible over the few months following treatment.

High dose

The neurotoxicity of the vinca alkaloids allows no significant dose escalation from standard doses.

INDEX